DYING FOR CARE:

Hospice Care or Euthanasia

"I hope we restore society's sense of the value of life. We must restore the joy in caring for people who are dying."

Dorothy C.H. Ley, MD, FRCP(C), FACP
Founder and Past President of the Canadian Palliative Care
Foundation

This book is dedicated to all the family members, friends, volunteers and health care professionals who provide the spirit and knowledge of hospice care to people who have a terminal or life-threatening illness. Hospice is not a place or a program but a philosophy of loving care. Those who practice this caring philosophy deserve our support and our gratitude.

This book is written with loving thanks to Janet Klees who encourages, supports and edits all my writing.

DYING FOR CARE:

Hospice Care or Euthanasia

HARRY VAN BOMMEL

NC Press Limited
Toronto, 1992

To contact author for speaking engagements, write or call:
PSD Consultants,
11 Miniot Circle
Scarborough, ON, Canada
M1K 2K1
(416) 264-4665

Canadian Cataloguing in Publication Data

van Bommel, Harry
  Dying for care

Includes bibliographical references and index.
ISBN 1-055021-073-4

I. Hospice care - Canada.
2. Hospices (Terminal care) - Canada.   I. Title
3. Euthanasia - Canada

R726.8.V35   1992   362.1'75   C92-093513-3

We would like to thank the Ontario Arts Council, the Ontario Publishing
Centre, the Ontario Ministry of Culture and Communications, and the Canada
Council for their assistance in the production of this book.

New Canada Publications, a division of NC Press Limited,
Box 452, Station A, Toronto, Ontario, Canada, M5W 1H8.

Printed and bound in Canada

CONTENTS

Author's Note   6
Acknowledgements   8
Introduction   11

Part 1: Hospice Care

Chapter 1   Living Fully Until Death:
Two Stories   15

Chapter 2   Canadian Palliative Care:
Meeting the Full Range of Human Needs   22

Chapter 3   Palliative Care
Within Our Flawed Health Care System   29

Chapter 4   Analysis of Palliative Care Today   35

Chapter 5   Standards of Care:
How Do We Get the Palliative Carc We Need?   46

Chapter 6   Reflections on Palliative Care:
Voices from the Front Line   52

Chapter 7   Palliative Care in the Year 2000:
What We Need to Do   58

Part 2: Euthanasia

Chapter 8   Euthanasia:
Common Arguments For and Against   69

Chapter 9   Euthanasia:
Voices from the Front Line   82

Chapter 10   Hospice Care or Euthanasia:
Personal Reflections   98

Bibliography   107
Index   110

AUTHOR'S NOTE

In writing a book on hospice care and euthanasia I was concerned with the needs of two different audiences who might read this book: the general public and people in the field of hospice care. I have chosen to concentrate first on people who can make decisions to improve Canadian hospice care locally, provincially and nationally. These people include members of the general public who already are interested in hospice care, hospice board members, professional and volunteer caregivers, government policy makers and people who fund hospice care. The book remains relevant, however, to all people interested in hospice care and euthanasia. The individual decisions we all make will ultimately have a great impact on the future of Canadian hospice care.

I have relied extensively on information provided by palliative caregivers and other experts in hospice care and euthanasia through questionnaires they answered. When reading their thoughts I recommend you also look up their names in the index so that you can read all of their other quotes in this book and put their comments into context.

In this book the terms palliative care and hospice care are both used to describe the active and loving supports (physical, emotional, spiritual and informational) given people who have a terminal or life-threatening illness. Both terms are used across Canada to represent care provided in the community, in hospitals, long term care facilities and in free-standing hospices.

Family is used throughout this book to include one's closest friends.

Patient and client are used throughout to mean anyone who has a terminal or life-threatening illness and who is receiving some kind of hospice care support.

People with a terminal illness refers to those who are generally expected to live less than six to twelve months. Life-threatening illness refers to such diseases as end-stage heart disease, AIDS, cancer, and some neuromuscular diseases. People with these life- threatening illnesses have periods where their lives may end unexpectedly due to complications but they are also likely to live relatively healthy lives for many years.

I would like to thank the Journal of Palliative Care for permission to reprint large portions of the following articles:

Roy, David J.
1990 "Euthanasia – Taking a Stand." *Journal of Palliative Care*. 6:(1):3-5.
1990 "Euthanasia – Where to Go After Taking a Stand." *Journal of Palliative Care*. 6:(2):3-5.

I would also like to thank Knoll Pharmaceuticals for permission to reproduce large portions of the following article for Chapter 5 of this book:

van Bommel, Harry
1991 "Palliative Care Standards – Who Decides?" *Pain Management Newsletter.* edited by Barry R. Ashpole. Markham, Ontario: Knoll Pharmaceuticals Canada. 4:(3):3-5.

ACKNOWLEDGEMENTS

Caroline Walker and Cathleen Kneen of NC Press have been instrumental in making sure this book was published. Their commitment to Canadian authors and social justice issues are a credit to the Canadian publishing industry. I also appreciate the encouragement given me by the members of the editorial board of NC Press during the development of this book. My thanks as well to Andrew Martindale, Kristen Thomson, and Winky Lai for turning the manuscript into a readable and widely distributed book.

I would like to thank Robert Shipley for his invaluable assistance. My thanks also to the Board and members of Trinity Hospice Toronto for their support and encouragement.

I wanted this book to reflect not just my own perspectives but also the wide range of opinions on the issues of hospice care and euthanasia in Canada. I sent questionnaires to some of Canada's leading palliative care practitioners (both professionals and volunteers) to get their thoughts and beliefs about hospice care and euthanasia. I am most grateful to those able to respond within the short time period they were given for their insights and for their efforts to help educate Canadians about these important issues. The expansion of Canadian hospice care and the euthanasia debate desperately need their opinions and perspectives. I feel privileged to read their compassion and commitment towards patients and families. I hope the readers will too. Their comments reflect their personal ideas and beliefs and do not necessarily reflect the policies of the organizations with which they are associated.

There were several anonymous submissions and I have respected their request for anonymity. My gratitude to them is just as real as to: **Heather M. Balfour,** Executive Director, Community Hospice Association (P.E.I.); **Laurie Bennett**, Executive Director, Hospice of Peel, Inc.; a group of Brockville, Ontario practitioners: **Janis Brown**, Palliative Care Consult Nurse; **Cheryl Chapman**, Community Outreach Co-ordinator; **Shirley Cooper**, Bereavement Co-ordinator; **Barbara Noonan**, Palliative Care Nurse Consultant; **Wilma O'Connell**, Palliative Care Program Director; **Gertrude Paul**, Palliative Care Consult Nurse; and **Sandra Thompson**, Palliative Care Consult Nurse; **Carol Derbyshire**, Executive Director, Hospice of Windsor; **Dr. Louis Dionne**, Director General of Maison Michel Sarrazin (Sillery, Quebec); **Rev. Sally Eaton**, Staff Chaplain, The Wellesley Hospital, Toronto; **Linda Gilpin**, R.N., Coordinator of Palliative Care, North York General Hospital; **Larry Grossman**, Physician Manager, Palliative Care Program, Scarborough Grace Hospital; **Joan Henderson**, President, Hospice King; **Elizabeth Latimer**, M.D., Director of Palliative Care, Hamilton Civic Hospital; **Dorothy C.H. Ley**, MD, FRCP(C), FACP, Founder and Past President of the Canadian Palliative Care Foundation; **Cecile Lynes**, Co-ordinator, Toronto Citizen Advocacy; **Evelyn MacKay**, former nurse, therapeutic touch practitioner, palliative care volunteer and teacher; **Jackie MacKenzie**, Executive Director, Hospice of London; **Tom Malcomson**, Professor, George Brown College and Member of the Southern Ontario Training Group; **Balfour Mount**, MD, FRCS(S), Professor of Palliative Medicine and Director of Palliative Care Medicine, McGill University; **Barbara O'Connor**, Executive Director, The Hospice of All Saints (Ottawa); **Joanne C. Oosterhuis-Giliam**, Clinical Director, Hopewell Children's Homes; **Catherine A. Rakchaev**, R.N., CEO, The Dorothy Ley Hospice; **David J. Roy**, BA(Math), STB, STL, PhL, Dr Theol, Director of the Center for Bioethics, Clinical Research Institute of Montreal; **Dr. Margaret R. Scott**, Associate Professor of Medicine, Memorial University of Newfoundland and Provincial Consultant, Palliative Care, Newfoundland Cancer Treatment and Research Foundation; **Marilynne Seguin**, Executive Director, Dying With Dignity; Trinity Hospice Toronto members: **Elaine Hall**, Resource Person; **Beth Pelton**, Co-ordinator; and **Pam Leeb**, Board Member; **Steven Waring**, Palliative Care Volunteer, Hospice Dufferin (Orangeville, Ontario); **Virginia Clark Weir**, Manager, Continuing and Palliative Care, Scarborough Grace Hospital; Wellington Hospice Members: **Walter Boos**, President; **Jackson E. Mathieue M.D.**, Medical Director; **Barbara Plunkett**, Coordinator; **Wolf Wolfensberger**, Professor, Syracuse University Division of Special Education and Rehabilitation, Director, Training Institute for Human Service Planning and developer of the PASSING Evaluation Tool for Human Services.

I would like to thank the following people for providing up-to-date information on federal, provincial and territorial government health plans for the next ten years: **Primrose Bishop**, Director, Hospital Services Division, Department of Health, Government of Newfoundland and Labrador; **Lynn Currie**, Lifestyle Educator, Department of Health and Fitness, Province of Nova Scotia; **Susi Derrah**, Senior Researcher, Premier's Council on Health Strategy, Province of New Brunswick; **M. Jane Fulton**, Ph.D., Professor of Strategic Management and Health Policy, University of Ottawa; **Joy Kajiwara**, Director, Continuing Care, Yukon Health and Social Services; **Bruno Lortie**, Political Counsellor, Ministry of Health; **Sylvia Mandryk**, RN, B.ScN., Policy Officer, Long Term Care/Rehabilitation Section, Community Health Division, Government of the Northwest Territories; **Sandra McKenzie**, Director, Community Health, Government of the Northwest Territories; **Diana Morrison**, Researcher, Cancer 2000; **Andre Nolet**, Consultant, Health Administration, Institutional and Professional Services, Health and Welfare Canada; **Anna Rose Spina**, Ontario Ministry of Health, Institutional Health Division, Policy and Support Unit; **Chris Tocher**, Health Information Line, Ministry of Health, Communications and Education, Province of British Columbia.

Several people helped review the first draft of this book. I am grateful for their insight, grammatical expertise and generosity of spirit. Their assistance has helped make this book more readable and useful. Any errors remain my own. My sincere thanks to: **Barry Ashpole, Kathy Bowden, Sally Eaton, Norman Endicott, Maureen Hennessy, Tom Malcomson, and Michael Roman.**

My thanks, as always, to **Janet Klees** for making it possible for me to take time off to write this book. Her encouragement, editorial suggestions and insights improve everything I write.

INTRODUCTION

For most people in North America the thought of killing themselves or having a family member, friend or doctor help them to die goes against their personal beliefs.

In 1991 the book *Final Exit* was published to help people who are dying understand the "practicalities of self-deliverance [suicide] and assisted suicide." The hard cover book sold over 500,000 its first year (20,000 copies in Canada). I believe the popularity of *Final Exit* is due to the real fear that North Americans have about dying in pain with tubes stuck in many parts of their bodies as they await the end in an intensive care unit or in a hospital ward. The publication of such a book demands a public response – not just to speak either for or against euthanasia, but to put euthanasia into the context of the needs of people who have a terminal or life-threatening illness. *Dying for Care* is one public response.

We must increase public awareness of all the choices available to people who are dying, especially the choice of hospice care. That is to say that we must increase the physical, emotional, spiritual and informational supports to make hospice care available to people across Canada.

My purpose in writing this book is to argue that euthanasia is not the way to meet the needs of people who are dying. The euthanasia movement sweeping this continent is a dangerous and ill-informed answer to the human realities and dilemmas of death and to the economic problems facing our health care system.

Derek Humphry, author of *Final Exit* and co-founder of the Hemlock Society in the United States, says that "Quality of life, personal dignity, self-control, and above all, choice, are what both hospice and the euthanasia movements are concerned with. . . . Both hospice and euthanasia provide valuable services to different types of people with varying problems" (p. 36-37). The difference between Humphry's book and this one is simple: *Final Exit* discusses the benefits of suicide and assisted suicide with three pages on hospice care; *Dying for Care* discusses the benefits and need for more hospice care and examines euthanasia within the greater context of what people who are dying really want. *Dying for Care* also presents current information on Canadian hospice care as well as providing a public forum for the thoughts of some of Canada's palliative care and euthanasia experts.

Across Canada there are people who have a terminal or life-threatening illness, such as the end stages of heart disease, cancer, and AIDS, who are pain free, mentally alert, able to participate in making decisions, and talk with their families, comfortable and able to give and receive emotional and spiritual support with the people they love. These people are benefiting from palliative care either through a formal program of care or through an informal network of support from their doctors, visiting home nursing, homecare programs, neighbours, and their families. Unfortunately they are not the majority.

This book is called *Dying for Care* because across Canada people are suffering needlessly before they die. They do not have the physical, emotional, spiritual and informational supports they should have. In fact, the palliative care movement is partly a response to a health care system that has not provided sufficient care for people who are dying.

The health care system in this country is among the best in the world. Our country's commitment to quality health care has given us a system with the resources, the skilled professionals and volunteers to provide excellent health care including palliative care to everyone. We have no excuse as a nation for tolerating the kind of pain and suffering that so many people endure before they die.

Managing pain is possible for over 90% of all patients with cancer when the proper methods are used. The World Health Organization, (WHO) with the help of experts from around the world (including Canada), has developed a simple protocol for managing pain and helping patients stay mentally alert. The WHO protocol uses commonly available medications to control pain. These medications are used for three main levels of pain: mild (non-narcotics, e.g. aspirin); moderate-severe (intermediate strength narcotic, e.g. codeine); and very severe pain (potent narcotic, e.g. morphine). Each doctor in Canada received this protocol through the federal health ministry, yet many doctors are reluctant to use the methods because they have little personal experience with them. Many family physicians have only one or two patients a year who have a terminal or life-threatening illness. Unless physicians begin to apply simple pain management, patients will continue to suffer needless pain or experience unnecessary drug-induced coma states.

Dying for Care is written in the hope that it will encourage public awareness and informed debate. The alternative is a public and political debate on the pros and cons of legalized euthanasia which will take away much needed energy and resources from palliative care. Such a debate would focus on the narrow issue of euthanasia and avoid looking at the larger context of how we value our own lives and the lives of others. Reducing everything to a pros-and-cons debate of the necessity of euthanasia would once again simplify a complex social issue into a legalistic argument that prevents all of us from making significant improvements in the lives of people across Canada. We must not fall into the trap of a debate on euthanasia that polarizes us and leads to bitterness and even resentment similar to what has happened during the abortion or capital punishment debates. We need an informed debate which will encourage people to work together to improve the lives of all Canadians.

If palliative care is not immediately expanded and improved across Canada, I fear that euthanasia will become a choice of desperation rather than education. If that happens it will not be because Canadians believe in euthanasia as the best method by which to die but rather that Canadians were not given the choice of palliative care (formal and informal) and therefore, not given acceptable life-affirming choices.

I once believed in the individual rights of people to choose assisted euthanasia for themselves. I no longer hold this belief. Helping my parents and grandfather to live at home until their deaths (between 1980-1984) helped me see euthanasia from the perspective of people who were dying. Researching hospice care and euthanasia over the past seven years gave me a greater understanding of the complex moral and political issues involved. However, it was not until I began struggling with writing this book that I was forced to examine, change and explain my beliefs in the greater context of making any life and death decision.

This book has been written to share these complexities and open the debate. In that spirit, I must begin by making clear my own perspective, my general values and those related specifically to hospice care and euthanasia.

1. I believe that all people deserve to receive, and give, spiritual, emotional, physical and informational support (the palliative care philosophy) at all times during their lives, not just at a time they have a terminal or life-threatening illness.

2. I believe that relationships are more important than policies, procedures or material things. I believe we need to spend more of our valuable time developing and enhancing our relationships with family, friends, colleagues, and other people who need our support. At the same time we must ensure that palliative care programs do not become bureaucratic to the point where individual patients no longer receive the spirit of the palliative care philosophy.

3. I believe a person's individual rights (e.g. making informed choices in life-and-death decisions) come with individual responsibilities (e.g. do no harm to others) which sometimes leads to moral dilemmas.

4. I believe that occasionally we must accept uncertainty on social issues (such as euthanasia) rather than risk inherent systemic abuses that can come from specific legislation, no matter how well written or well intended.

Specifically in relation to hospice care and euthanasia:

1. I believe that we must increase the number and quality of informal and formal palliative care programs across Canada.

2. I believe that our emphasis on euthanasia is taking away valuable time, efforts and resources from expanding and improving palliative care.

3. I believe we should not legalize euthanasia.

The book is divided into two sections: Part 1 – the history, importance, and need for expanded and improved hospice care; Part 2 – the euthanasia debate including thoughts from palliative care experts. The last chapter presents my own conclusions.

My view on euthanasia has not prevented me, I hope, from presenting a balanced view on that issue in Part 2 of this book. I hope this book presents some of the complexity of this issue and the struggle each of us must go through to come up with our own answers.

The main point, however, remains the desperate needs of people who have a terminal or life-threatening illness. They need the spirit and knowledge of palliative care through informal or formal programs.

CHAPTER 1

LIVING FULLY UNTIL DEATH: TWO STORIES

Palliative care is the physical, emotional, spiritual and informational support given to someone who has a terminal or life-threatening illness and to their families. The following are the stories of Mary and Frank's illness and their deaths. Mary's story is somewhat typical of how many people die in Canada today. Frank's story represents the hospice approach to living life fully until you die. Some of the details of these composite stories have been changed to respect people's privacy.

Mary

In 1974 Mary's family doctor found a lump in Mary's breast. After several tests and visits to various doctors Mary had a radical mastectomy to remove her left breast. Her husband Sam and three children (Susan, Pat and Bob) were very supportive even though they were not always sure of how to help Mary.

A year after her mastectomy Mary began to feel an intense, piercing pain in her chest. She thought her cancer may be returned and her gripping anxiety worsened the pain. Mary's son Bob was home from university and got Mary to agree to go to her local hospital Emergency Department for tests and possible treatments. Her cancer specialists did several tests to discover if her cancer had spread. Mary's doctors took her husband, Sam, aside and told him that Mary may have pulled a muscle in her chest and there was nothing to worry about. There was no cancer visible in any of her tests. They suggested that Mary's worry about her cancer coming back was common in women who have had a mastectomy and that Sam just needed to be extra supportive a little while longer. The doctors told Sam that Mary would receive physiotherapy for her chest pain "just in case she really did pull a muscle."

Mary's pain did not reduce with the physiotherapy. After two months of hot and cold treatments for her 'muscle strain', Mary's condition continued to worsen over the Christmas holidays. She ended up in bed for most of the holidays feeling increased chest pain, fatigue and stomach upset. One morning, soon after Christmas, Sam found Mary unconscious on their bedroom floor. It appeared she had tried to get to the bathroom on her own and had collapsed. Sam called 911 and Mary was rushed to hospital. She was in a coma and Sam was told she might not live through the day.

Mary's children flew in from various cities across Canada. The swiftness of the change in their mother's condition traumatised them and many of the subsequent days are just a blur in their memories today.

Mary recovered from her coma after several days. Her doctors told her very little but did tell Sam that there was nothing more they could do for Mary. They had discovered that her cancer had returned and was now present in her brain, liver, lungs, the sac around her heart and in her bones. The pain in her chest must have been bone cancer all along but had not shown up on X-rays only a few months before. The doctors were genuinely upset that they had not caught the cancer early enough. They were visibly saddened by Mary's condition and wished her family luck in caring for Mary at home.

Mary lived at home for a few months during which time Sam told her that her cancer had spread and that she had only a short time to live. Mary and Sam shared tears and love during that and subsequent talks. They were each other's best friend and their 30 years of marriage was coming to an end. The children were with their parents and shared in the practical and emotional care of their mother. There were times when Mary comforted her children, as she had done so many times before, and times when Susan, Patricia and Bob comforted her.

Mary's pain continued to increase and the pain medication she was on was clearly not working. One night at 2:30 a.m. Mary sat bolt up in bed and begged her family and God to let her die. She began reciting The Lord's Prayer loudly in hopes that her pain would subside. After a time she went on her hands and knees in bed and rocked back and forth with low pitched moans to try and reduce the pain.

Mary's family doctor came within the hour and gave her morphine.

For the next two weeks Mary was in and out of semi-consciousness and was expected to die at any moment. When the family could no longer deal with the poorly managed physical pain Mary was suffering at home and their own emotional strain, they had Mary transferred to the hospital. Mary was, in fact, only a few days away from her death. Her admittance to hospital through the Emergency Department led to aggressive treatment of her condition. At one point it was determined, without consulting the family, that Mary's condition was worsening much too quickly and that she needed to go on a respirator if she was to continue to live. Mary had discussed this possibility with her family and had asked them to avoid life-support techniques if she was near death anyway.

Mary remained on a respirator for another two weeks. Her family went mostly without sleep and began to feel that they had failed Mary. They stayed with her round-the-clock since no one could say when she might awaken from her drug-induced coma or die. After much soul searching the family asked that Mary's life-support be removed. Her doctors had done some further tests and agreed with their decision. They made it clear to the family that there was no reason to keep Mary on life-support since her cancer was overtaking most of her body. After several more days of discussions and waiting, Mary was given heavy sedation and her life-support systems were withdrawn. Mary died a short time later.

Sam, Susan, Patricia and Bob still have nightmares about Mary's last few months. There are so many questions unanswered. Why had Mary's cancer not been stopped after her mastectomy? Why had her cancer spread so quickly a year later? Why was her chest pain not investigated more carefully? Why were there not more supports available to Mary and her family so that she could stay at home as she had wanted? Why was her family not consulted about her treatment, especially the use of life-support systems? Why had the family not known more about how to help Mary? What would they do without Mary as the centre of their home? What would become of Sam with the children going back to their own homes in other cities?

It has been 17 years since Mary's death. She is still very much in the minds and hearts of her family. Patricia is now a palliative care nurse. She and her family wish that the spirit and knowledge of palliative care had been available to them in 1975 – the year palliative care officially began in Canada.

Frank

Frank was a middle-aged construction worker who had worked for 25 years for the same company. Together with his wife, June, and his two children Elizabeth and Bill, they have lived in the same modest bungalow for the last 19 years.

In 1989 Frank finally went for a medical check-up. Frank did not trust doctors and had avoided seeing one for several years. However he had begun to feel more tired at work and was easily out of breath so June had convinced him to see their family doctor. The doctor discovered some difficulties with Frank's lungs. Although Frank had begun a few years before to smoke less than his usual two-packs of cigarettes a day it seems that his lungs were irreparably damaged. After further tests it was confirmed that Frank had lung cancer.

Frank went through various treatments of chemotherapy which stopped the cancerous growth for a time. The treatments were physically difficult for him but the hope of improving his health was worth the risks his doctors had fully described to him. His family worried about Frank but also changed some of their schedules to make sure that they could provide physical and emotional support to Frank while allowing him to continue to fulfill his role as father and husband. In other words, they didn't treat Frank like an invalid and if they did occasionally slip into a maternal behaviour he reminded them that he was still the Frank he always was, except that now he was also struggling to overcome his cancer.

Later in 1990 the cancer began to spread and the pain forced Frank back into hospital. After more tests, Frank's doctors told him that there were no other medical things they could do to cure him. They assured him that they would continue to care for him since their primary role now was to help Frank enjoy his life as fully as possible. This support included pain management that helped Frank remain relatively pain free and mentally alert.

When the doctors thought the time was right, a few days after they controlled Frank's pain and other symptoms, they told Frank about the palliative care program in the hospital which was available to him and his family. The professionals and volunteers in this program would provide as much physical, emotional, and spiritual supports as Frank and his family would like. The doctors told him that these supports could increase or decrease over time since Frank would choose the supports he and his family wanted.

Frank was given some written information about the palliative care program and a short list of books and articles that might provide further information. They promised to answer any and all of his questions honestly and in as much detail as he asked for.

His family learned about the palliative care program from Frank. They were still adjusting to the idea that Frank might die within six months and were not immediately interested in the idea of having more strangers enter their lives. They took the written material about the program home but didn't begin to read it until Frank was scheduled to return home from the hospital.

Before Frank returned to his bungalow (colourfully decorated to welcome "Dad" home) the Home Care Coordinator in the hospital arranged for daily nurses' visits. She also ordered a hospital bed to make it easier for the family to help Frank who was now bedridden most of the time.

Over the next few months Frank's family and friends took turns being with him. Frank sometimes felt frightened about the future and other times felt blessed to have his family and friends so close by. These times were spent laughing, crying, remembering, planning and just being quiet together. Frank's pain and other symptoms were well controlled. He was physically comfortable and mentally alert. The daily nursing visits were switched to three times a week for several months as Frank didn't need the daily care. In time his physical condition did require more care and the daily visits were started again.

In Frank's last few weeks he was given the choice of remaining at home or going into the hospital's palliative care unit. In the unit his family could concentrate on being with Frank rather than on providing most of his physical care. His family could still bring home-cooked meals, special photographs and other items from home that would help make Frank feel comfortable.

Frank, June, Elizabeth and Bill discussed the alternatives of Frank staying at home or going to the palliative care unit at the hospital. Frank worried about the extra work his staying at home would cause June and the children. Elizabeth and Bill were able to take some time away from school to be with their parents most of the times. At the same time they were able to keep up with most of their studies when other family members and friends came to visit. The school had been very understanding and flexible with their homework assignments.

June, Elizabeth and Bill told Frank they wanted him to stay at home. They recognized the advantages of the hospital but felt that they could take better care of him at home with the help of Home Care's visiting nurses, the help of a visiting homemaker (a person who helps with cleaning, cooking, and shopping arranged through Home Care), and the help of other family, friends and neighbours.

With the support of his family physician and Home Care, Frank's life at home was well supported with compassion and the love of his family and friends. The Palliative Care Program at the hospital provided information to help the family learn how they could support Frank at home and what to expect as his illness progressed. There were difficult times of trying to say goodbye mixed with the love of family and friends "being there" for him. Frank remained mentally alert till the day before his death. Slowly over his last few weeks he found he needed more and more sleep. The day before his death he went to sleep and died peacefully at home the next day. His priest had been to see him several times during his illness and returned on the day he died to provide support to his family.

Frank's family misses his strength, humour, and his loving hugs. They feel that they did the best they could for Frank and are proud that their support allowed Frank to live his life as fully as possible under the circumstances. They remember the months before his death as both sad and happy because they, as a family, were open about their fears, anxiety and love. There were few things left unsaid.

Frank suffered the loss of his job and future. His death was not a Hollywood fantasy where everything went perfectly well. There were the typical bureaucratic problems with getting the necessary professional supports, equipment and medications. There were days of doubt and anger. But there was also time to prepare to say his goodbyes to family and friends. There was time to make the legal, financial and funeral arrangements without a mad rush. There was time to explore unresolved issues and some of those (not all) were resolved.

Comparison of the Two Stories

In both cases Mary and Frank received the loving support of their families. This is not always typical in Canada where so many women outlive their husbands, and where many people have no family or friends nearby at all. In both stories it was obvious that Mary and Frank's lives until they died were not picture perfect. Mary did not receive the palliative care that Frank received. Mary's case is more typical of our current situation in Canada. In Sutherland and Fulton's 1988 book, *Health Care in Canada*, they estimate the 95% of Canadians do not receive palliative care. Frank's case, however, is not a fairy tale and good Canadian models of hospice care do exist across Canada.

The problem is, there is not enough support for people who are dying and their families. Let us look at Mary's story.

There was:
- little direct communication between patient and doctors
- Mary's description of her chest pain was minimized
- her family was poorly prepared to provide the physical and emotional support she needed
- both Mary and her family had little information to help them know what to do and what to expect
- Mary's pain and symptoms were not well controlled
- there was inadequate home care available including night-time nursing care
- life-support systems were used without discussions
- no bereavement follow-up was offered to help the family answer their many questions

---

These are the very points that palliative care was developed to change.

In Frank's story there was open communication between all the various people involved in his care. Frank and his family were in charge of most of the decision making. The hospital palliative care program provided information to help Frank and his family know what to do and what to expect. Frank's pain and other symptoms were well managed. While there was no bereavement follow-up by the hospital it appears that their family priest provided the support the family needed.

Now that we have seen some of the practical supports that palliative care can provide patients and families let us examine Canadian palliative care more closely.

CHAPTER 2

CANADIAN PALLIATIVE CARE: MEETING THE FULL RANGE OF HUMAN NEEDS

As we have seen in Chapter 1, there is a huge difference between dying without palliative care (Mary's story) or with it (Frank's story). The palliative care philosophy (also called hospice care) is an old one of caring for people who are dying. Understanding the various palliative care models available in Canada now will help us understand what is necessary in the future.

Palliative care is the active and loving care given to people who have a life-threatening or terminal illness and to their families. It provides physical, emotional, spiritual and informational supports to help improve the quality of a person's remaining life, and recognizes the patient and family as the principal decision makers.

Dorothy C.H. Ley, MD, FRCP(C), FACP, founder and past president of the Canadian Palliative Care Foundation and present Chair of the Dorothy Ley Hospice in Etobicoke, Ontario, in her keynote address at the 1991 Canadian Palliative Care Conference in Vancouver, said:

"Palliative care began in Canada in the institutional setting with the development of palliative care units. The Canadian health care system has consistently under-funded and underemphasized the community as a site for care. These two phenomena led to the establishment of many voluntary community based programs and to home care and community nursing organizations incorporating palliative care into their services. The result has been a patchwork of highly motivated, innovative hospice programs. Unfortunately, most are poorly funded and lack sufficient professional staff to provide the interdisciplinary care to which they subscribe."

Palliative care provides a model of holistic care with either some, or all, of the following people being involved in giving interdisciplinary care: family members and friends; family doctors; community clergy; palliative care doctors, nurses, chaplains, social workers; pharmacists; dieticians; occupational and physio therapists; art and music therapists; masseurs; psychologists and psychiatrists; homemakers and volunteers. There should, however, rarely be a situation when all of these people are involved with someone who has a terminal or life-threatening illness. We must avoid the potential danger of a fully-integrated palliative care system where too many people are involved with someone in the last stage of their life. People need security, comfort and compassion with some practical assistance from different caregivers. A program with too many professionals may require patients to receive services they may not want, or need, in order to fully utilize the services of paid staff. This is one of the dilemmas of our high-cost, medical-model health care system where increasingly people require more and more services simply because those services exist. It is one of the reasons why parts of our health care system still perceive maternity care, aging and dying as diseases requiring professional services.

In contrast to the technological methods of today's advanced health care system, palliative care represents a return to a more humane, patient-oriented philosophy of care that encourages patients, their families, and their caregivers to work together. Palliative care can be provided at home, in a hospital, in a long term care facility, in a special palliative care unit in a hospital, or in a free-standing hospice centre. Palliative care may occasionally use high technology to help manage a patient's pain or symptoms but this technology acts as a supplement to the person's care. In acute care hospitals this relationship is often reversed where "care" is secondary to the technological/pharmaceutical focus on "cure."

Hospice care and palliative care are the same thing. In Great Britain and the U.S.A. the word "hospice" is used most often. Hospice in French means dying in the poorhouse so the term "palliative care" was preferred in Canada in the mid-1970s. Both terms are now used across Canada. There is a trend in Canada to refer to the care given in hospitals as palliative care and care given in the community as hospice care. This trend is dangerous because some people use the different terms to imply that one form of palliative care may be better than another, which is not true. When a system of care assumes that patients and family have the primary role in decision-making, then the system must allow for different methods and places of providing palliative care.

The holistic palliative model should not be limited to people who are dying. Anyone who has ever stayed in a hospital will understand that they too need physical, emotional, spiritual and informational support to varying degrees.

Philosophy of Palliative Care

Hospice care is as much a philosophy as it is a program or an institution. There is an image of dying people that many Canadians have – the person is comatose, hooked up to monitors with intravenous tubes sticking out everywhere. We have too often seen our loved ones like this and we have seen them in pain and suffering.

Hospice care is different. It makes sure that someone is relatively free of pain, is often able to be awake so they can remain an active part of their families until a few hours or days before death, does not use monitors or tubes, and tries to give as much control to the patient and family as they choose to have.

The practical elements of hospice care are more fully discussed in my book *Choices for People Who Have a Terminal Illness, Their Families and Their Caregivers*. I have summarized a few key points here for reference only.

The goal of hospice care is not to cure an illness nor to prolong life heroically. Surgical procedures are recommended only if they help a patient's physical comfort. Few tests are carried out unless they, too, can improve a patient's comfort. Even in communities where there is no official hospice care program, neighbours, family physicians, clerics and friends work together as a team to help someone in need. In fact, Trinity Hospice Toronto has established a community hospice program built upon helping people set up such teams for themselves rather than working within a formal palliative care program.

Once pain and other symptoms of an illness are under control, the patient and family have time to spend on their emotional, spiritual and informational needs. A major concern of patients and families is what the death will be like. According to palliative care experts, proper pain and symptom control in cancer patients, for example, permits the person to be alert and communicative until a short time before they die. They often slip into unconsciousness and die in the way most of us would like, in their sleep.

There are specific ways to help patients and families. Generally, emotional support means active listening. Such listening can be done by any and all of the caregivers and includes having the patient and family actively involved in the decision-making process. It means providing them with the information they ask for and helping them learn effective communication skills so that their hopes and needs are met as well as possible.

Helping patients and families spiritually does not necessarily require a chaplain, priest, pastor, or rabbi. It may be as simple as listening to patients' thoughts, beliefs and fears of dying, of an afterlife, or of a review of their lives in search for meaning. This spiritual element is often missing when we care for people who are dying and yet it can be the most comforting and hopeful form of caring.

Informational support means providing people with understandable information. It may be spoken, written down, video or audiotaped, or presented in group discussions. People have different informational needs. Some people want only very basic information, while others want volumes of information to help them decide what is best. People only remember about 20% of what they hear or read and they forget most of that within 24 hours. Therefore, information must come in different packages to allow them to return to the information when they need it most, often when no one else is around.

A major benefit to hospice care is that rules are kept to a minimum. The more organized the palliative care program the more rules there will be. Clients and families may want palliative care programs that are informal or formal. Choosing a program depends on the availability of different types of programs in a community and how soon a patient and family become aware of their choices.

The other major benefit of hospice care is that the professional and volunteer caregivers also receive support. So often in institutions the caregivers have little opportunity to discuss their feelings, concerns and hopes for their patients. When a patient dies caregivers often have no time to discuss the loss. In effective hospice care the caregivers are encouraged and given time to talk to their colleagues, to learn from each other and to share the losses they feel. Staff turnover in hospice care is very low relative to other forms of health care. I believe this is, in great part, because the professional and volunteer caregivers are able to give more of themselves to their patients and receive more in return.

Different Types of Care

The following is a list of the various types of hospice care available in Canada. Different communities choose different models based on their needs and the funds they are able to raise.

1) **Home care and community hospices:** caring for someone at home is often the key component of hospice care programs. These programs may be funded and coordinated by a provincial government or affiliated with a specific hospital, palliative care unit or coordinated through public health agencies as a hospice outreach program. Sometimes home care is strictly a community response to a need and is coordinated through a volunteer community hospice organization. In some communities the home care program is the only hospice care component available. With home care, the patient remains at home until death, rather than in a hospital or nursing home and is treated by visiting doctors, nurses, therapists, the clergy, and other caregivers. Principles of pain and symptom control, emotional, spiritual and informational support are followed.

In all hospice programs, home care is often considered the most important component because people who are dying are usually most comfortable in their own environment. Only in situations when the family and professional caregivers are unable to provide quality care would patients go to the hospital or, if available, a hospice care facility. Some patients, however, may choose to stay or go to their local hospital because they are more comfortable there. The hospice philosophy is about making that choice possible as well.

People receiving care at home may sometimes go to the hospital or free-standing hospice to get help with pain and symptom control. Once the pain or symptoms are managed the person returns home. Some home care programs, hospitals and free-standing hospices provide what is called "respite care" which allows a patient to stay there for a few days or weeks so that the family caregivers have a little time off from the 24-hour per day care many of them provide.

2) **Free-standing Hospices:** a facility separate from any other institution providing only hospice care (for example, Maison Michel Sarrazin in Sillery, Quebec and Casey House in Toronto). Patients are often referred by a family physician or by a specialist seeing the patient in a hospital. Depending on the resources of such a facility there may be space available in emergency situations. These facilities do not have operating rooms, specialized life-support systems or other features of a

regular hospital. At present there are only a handful of such hospices in Canada and most are affiliated with a nearby hospital.

3) **Palliative Care Units in a Hospital:** a separate unit within a hospital which provides all the services of a free-standing hospice except that patients are within easy access of hospital personnel and facilities. Because it is relatively easy to change part of hospital into a palliative care unit, such units are less expensive to begin than a free-standing facility. These units are often designed and decorated to give a more home-like atmosphere than other hospital units.

4) **Palliative Care Team (Consultation Team) within a Hospital:** rather than having a separate unit within a hospital, many hospitals now have a multi-disciplinary team of doctors, nurses and other caregivers who provide care to patients regardless where they are located in the hospital. This team often instructs the nurses and other caregivers throughout the hospital about how to provide palliative care. The team educates the regular caregivers in pain and symptom control and encourages the emotional, spiritual and informational supports that individual patients need. Hospitals with limited resources or those wishing to test the hospice philosophy may begin with a palliative care team. Other hospitals choose this model for philosophical reasons believing that patients should not be moved from the area where they are best known by the medical and nursing staff to a special unit somewhere else in the hospital. In this way all hospital staff would ideally become involved in palliative care, thereby advancing the concept throughout the organization. The palliative care team is usually very small (e.g. a full-time coordinator who is often a nurse, and part-time physicians, chaplains and social workers). Other professionals are brought in on an irregular basis. Volunteers may be recruited to help the patients, families and team members.

5) **Extended Care Services:** hospice programs in institutions such as nursing homes and long term care hospitals. These facilities may have a palliative care team and/or a special unit for patients who are dying.

6) **Regional Palliative Care Programs:** some regions of Canada, e.g. Victoria, B.C. and Ottawa-Carleton, Ontario have regionalized their palliative care programs to coordinate the services of hospital-based and community based hospice programs.

Conclusion

The philosophy of palliative care encourages a relaxation of the limits normally found in hospitals and long-term care facilities. Patients, family members, professional caregivers and volunteers work together, with a minimum of rules, to help patients live as full and complete lives as possible until their death. There is time for joy and hopefulness and a time for sadness and goodbyes. Palliative care has its difficulties. There will never be perfection in any palliative care model of care. The palliative care philosophy, however, provides us with the best guidelines to meet the needs of people who are dying while also providing support to their families and their caregivers.

CHAPTER 3

PALLIATIVE CARE WITHIN OUR FLAWED HEALTH CARE SYSTEM

This chapter examines the proposed governmental directions for health care in Canada in the next decade, the commitment of provincial and federal governments to palliative care, plus information about how our health care system does not treat all of us fairly. The chapter ends with a review of health care statistics.

Palliative care cannot be provided in a vacuum. It must be looked at in the context of the health care system in which people who are dying are being treated right now. They need either palliative care within hospitals and other health care facilities or they need early referral to palliative care services in the community. If, however, we as a society are to make informed decisions about palliative care, we need to understand the present health care situation in Canada.

General Canadian Health Strategies for Improving Our Health

Although provincial governments are planning for changes in palliative care there is still a lack of political commitment to act on the recommendations of the many recent health care reports. In some provinces the homecare and community health programs are grossly under-funded and uncoordinated. The development of over 300 palliative care programs in Canada by committed community and hospital leaders is a direct response to this lack of political leadership and funding in the health and social services ministries or departments.

Health care is the responsibility of the ten provinces and two territories in Canada. The federal government provides funds for some of the costs of health care in Canada and has a federal act to ensure relative equality of national health care. However, health care policies and funding remains primarily a provincial and territorial responsibility.

In the past ten years most, if not all, of the provinces and territories have re-examined their health care strategies. There has been a definite shift in emphasis from hospital treatment of illness to an emphasis on preventive medicine and treating people in their homes as much as possible.

Various provinces have come up with innovative proposals and programs to help meet the needs of patients who are chronically ill or who have a life-threatening or terminal illness.

In New Brunswick the government established a "hospital without walls." This Extra-Mural Hospital was established in 1981 as a "planned response to a combination of forces which were putting pressure on the health care system and which taken together may well have had the potential to overwhelm it. The factors which led to this hospital were: growth of population, high cost of construction of hospitals and other care institutions, high daily costs of keeping patients in institutions particularly in sophisticated high-technology hospitals, over-emphasis on institutionalization which developed after World War II, the changing pattern of disease (a shift to more long-term degenerative conditions away from short-term episodes of illness), and the aging of the population."

This hospital without walls is a community-based alternative to institutional care. Doctors admit and discharge patients to this homecare program as if they were patients in a hospital. Nurses, therapists, social workers, dieticians and others visit the patient at home to prevent people from having to go to hospital or to return them home sooner. Another goal is to help seniors avoid admission to nursing homes (either short or long term). The hospital also recognizes the invaluable help that loved ones provide to patients in their homes. They cite a British report which estimated that if loved ones no longer cared for the elderly at home it would cost an extra 5.3 billion pounds to the British health care system.

The province of Ontario is also looking at ways to improve the coordination of health care and social services. There is a proposed shift to: health promotion and disease prevention; fostering strong and supportive families and communities; ensuring a safe, high quality physical environment; increasing the number of years of good health for the citizens of Ontario by reducing illness, disability and premature death; and providing accessible, affordable, appropriate health services for all. The provision of palliative care is seen as a continuation of providing health and social services. The implementation and funding policies to make palliative care truly a part of the continuum of care have not been developed yet even though recommendations to do so have been part of government reports for many years.

Many provinces promote palliative care as part of their continuing care programs. In Nova Scotia, for example, the 1990 *Health Strategy for the Nineties* report discusses the necessity for improved co-ordination and integration of the health and community services needed by people with a terminal illness.

According to Sandra McKenzie, Director of Community Health in the Northwest Territories, palliative care is an integrated part of home care, long term care and hospital based services. The extent to which palliative care can be provided at home varies with the family's ability to provide support, the degree of nursing care required and the length of time involved. Another consideration is the many small communities spread out geographically across the territories. It is difficult to provide all the necessary services to every community but many are successfully provided in a linked system of support. This linked system includes 48 health centres and six hospitals as well as the physicians' offices and continuing care programs.

In British Columbia the 1991 *Report of The Royal Commission on Health Care and Costs* recommended some innovative strategies for changing the provincial health care systems. For example, it recommends that patients and their loved ones who provide care at home participate more actively in decisions about what type of home support should be provided and who will provide it. It further recommends that family members might be paid as home care workers in appropriate situations to help offset the costs of professionals providing care at home.

Specifically for palliative care, the B.C. report recommends programs in each community be coordinated, if possible, by volunteers working in partnership with local hospital and home care programs. These programs should include uniform guidelines, assured access to home nursing and home support, immediate access to community hospital beds, transfer of a portion of existing hospital and home care program budgets and the selection of palliative care teams from existing care providers and volunteers. Furthermore, the province would provide drugs, supplies, equipment and services necessary for in-home palliative care at no cost to the patients.

Our Health Care System Does Not Treat All of Us Fairly

The palliative care philosophy is patient-family centred and designed to meet the personal, cultural, and religious needs of individual patients and families. Our health care system, in general, recognizes diverse needs but is incapable of meeting those needs because of the immense size and complexity of the various provincial systems. Palliative care is, at present, a simpler and more flexible model of care, and can, therefore, avoid some of the inequities of our present health care system.

To understand why palliative care is necessary it is important to understand some of the problems of unequal treatment of people inherent within our health care system.

Cancer 2000 is a federal government-funded Canadian Cancer Society effort to look at the future of cancer care in Canada. One of the many reports presented to the Cancer 2000 initiative was submitted by the Members of the Panel on Cancer and the Disadvantaged. They concluded that "factors such as socioeconomic status, education, place of living, gender, age, mental or physical handicap and ethnocultural background, as well as one's genes, have been shown to produce inequalities in many areas of health." The limited information they were able to find on the inequalities of care in Canada confirmed that inequalities in care do exist especially for older people, aboriginal peoples, women in general, poor people and some ethnocultural communities.

In the introduction to their report they wrote about the widely held belief that universal health care systems like the ones in Canada and Britain would "lead to a narrowing of the gap in health status between the rich and the poor." This belief was shattered in Great Britain at least by the publication in 1980 of *The Black Report*, the report of the Working Group on Inequalities in Health. They concluded that people at the bottom of the social scale had much higher death rates. This was true regardless of age. In 1988 Margaret Whitehead confirmed these findings. Canadian studies have similar results (see J. Epp, 1986; National Council of Welfare, 1990).

Our health care system does not treat all of us fairly. Women, immigrants who do not speak English well (or French in Quebec), people with disabilities, elderly Canadians and aboriginal people are all at risk of not receiving the same degree of care as white, middle and upper-class men. Palliative care faces similar difficulties but its simpler and more flexible model has a greater likelihood of meeting the diverse needs of individual and family needs. At present, however, most of the people served are white, middle-class, English speaking (francophones in Quebec) Canadians. Most of the professional caregivers and volunteers I see at palliative care conferences are also from this same group of people. We are not yet meeting the needs of most people who have a terminal or life-threatening illness in Canada but the hospice care philosophy is the best model to date to address their needs.

How Many of Us Are Dying and Why

How many people die in Canada every year? What are they dying from? How many people receive palliative care?

According to Statistics Canada there were 26,833,000 people living in Canada in 1991. The most recent statistics available (1988) show that 190,011 people died that year, with between 70- 80% of them dying in hospitals.

The following list tells us what people died of during 1988:

57,861	heart disease	(30.45%)
50,756	cancer	(26.71%)
13,450	stroke	(7.08%)
15,979	respiratory disease	(8.41%)
9,436	accidents [4,355 in motor vehicles]	(4.97%)
3,492	suicides	(1.845%)
39,037	other	(20.54%)

More recent information gives us figures up to 1990 for people with AIDS: 5,010 reported AIDS cases, and 3,180 deaths.

Dr. Ralph Sutherland and Jane Fulton estimate in their 1988 book, *Health Care in Canada*, that less than five percent of dying people in Canada receive palliative care through formal recognized palliative care programs. They further estimate that perhaps 10% of cancer patients may receive palliative care. If we take these estimates as accurate then about 5,000-7,000 people received palliative care in 1988 most of whom had cancer. That means that over 100,000 people died with a terminal or life-threatening illness without receiving palliative care through a program. Furthermore the vast majority of people with end-stage heart disease, strokes, respiratory illness, and neuromuscular illnesses are not receiving palliative care at present in Canada. Some may have received palliative care in spirit (either at home or in hospital) but the vast majority would not have received the various supports they needed.

Across Canada our health care system and governments are identifying the need for more palliative care. However, there is very little political will to make the necessary changes. Our flawed health care system continues to treat people unfairly – not intentionally, perhaps – but because of the size, complexity, and inappropriate allocation of resources within the system. So the physical, emotional, spiritual and informational supports that patients and family need remain unmet. Less than five percent of Canadians are receiving hospice care similar to Frank's care (see Chapter 1). Some others receive elements of hospice care through their family and community supports. Many more, however, run the risk of Mary's scenario (also in Chapter 1). Is it any wonder that euthanasia, which provides a quick and controlled end, is so popular when the alternative for so many people is uncontrolled pain and mismanaged symptom control? What is clearly needed is more palliative care both through formal community and hospital programs and through informal hospice care provided at home.

The point is not to institutionalize or to spend billions of dollars providing unwanted services to people who are dying. The point is to provide supports to those who are dying and their families. The point is to give them back control over their lives just as they had before they became sick.

CHAPTER 4

ANALYSIS OF PALLIATIVE CARE TODAY

We have seen that there is not enough hospice care available in Canada. Although specific statistics are not available as yet it is easy to see that 345 programs across all of Canada cannot meet the needs of over 100,000 people who have a terminal or life-threatening illness. When you add a rough estimate of five family members per patient there are about a half a million people who may want either formal or informal palliative care at any one time. Most of these people do not know that palliative care exists and therefore do not ask for it. Palliative care at present in Canada is generally limited to patients with cancer or AIDS and most of those 55,000 people are also not getting sufficient palliative care. Those who do receive referrals to palliative care programs are often referred too late and have already suffered needlessly. Those who do receive the full benefits of informal and formal palliative care are the best spokespeople for the movement, yet we rarely ask them to speak on behalf of hospice care.

The following statistics of hospice care programs in Canada come from the latest *Canadian Palliative Care Directory*, 1990 edition. Included in this directory is a list of most provincial palliative care associations and full descriptions of programs available across Canada. The number and type of palliative care programs across Canada change every year. Some are cut because of budget restraints while elsewhere new ones begin. Some are run within the health care system while others are community based and raise funds like all not-for-profit organizations must do in Canada.

You can find out about hospice programs in your area by checking with your phone book, provincial palliative care association, local hospital, family doctor, church/synagogue/temple, homecare program or city/provincial government.

If you do not want to use a palliative care program or if there is not one available in your area you can form your own support team with the help of your family doctor, homecare, and your friends and neighbours. June Callwood in *Twelve Weeks in Spring* describes how one woman, Margaret Frazer, had a support team to allow her to stay at home until she died. In the 1992 edition of my book *Choices* there is a chapter on how to organize your own support team as well.

Analysis of Hospice Care Programs

The following statistics show the distribution of palliative care programs across Canada in 1990.

Table 1.

Alberta:	25 programs
British Columbia:	63 programs
Manitoba:	10 programs
New Brunswick:	11 programs
Newfoundland:	8 programs
Nova Scotia:	20 programs
Ontario:	143 programs
Prince Edward Island:	5 programs
Quebec:	41 programs
Saskatchewan:	18 programs
Yukon:	1 program
Northwest Territories:	no separately identified program
Total	345

The programs listed in table 1 do not include AIDS Committees that provide palliative care because that information is not yet available. Nor do the figures include informal or beginning programs that did not make the last (1990) edition of the directory.

Of the programs listed 38% are in the major provincial cities and 62% in smaller cities or towns/regions. Many palliative care programs began when people in an area decided that more care was needed for people who had a terminal or life-threatening illness. Community palliative care organizations evolved mostly in smaller communities rather than big cities. In larger cities palliative care was often begun on the initiative of medical caregivers within a hospital system.

Some of these programs help both adults and children but most concentrate on adults. Some services provide 24-hour care. Some provide bereavement support to family members after the death of a loved one. As noted earlier, different programs include some or all of the following members: nurses, doctors, pastors, social workers, volunteers, physiotherapists, occupational therapists, psychologists, pharmacists, dieticians, music and art therapists, and educational coordinators. These people may work full time for the program or work when needed.

These programs are located in hospitals, in long-term care facilities (e.g. nursing homes, chronic care hospitals), and in a free standing hospice (only 3-4 available in Canada to date). In a hospital there may be a palliative care team that comes to the patient anywhere in the hospital and/or they may have a special palliative care unit.

There has actually been a decrease in the number of programs in Canada from 1986 to 1990. In the report to Cancer 2000 Task Force by the Expert Panel on Palliative Care the following statistical analysis was presented. In 1986 the Canadian Palliative Care Foundation surveyed programs and found a total of 359. In 1990 that number is down to 345 with Alberta losing the most (down from 42 to 25). There has been an increase in community hospice programs (from 84 in 1986 to 105 in 1990) and a decrease in hospital-based programs (from 150 to 114). More hospital palliative care programs have been transferred to long-term care facilities (24% in 1990 versus 6% in 1986). Home care programs in existing community agencies now equal 48% of the total programs. There has been an increase in designated palliative care beds from 588 in 67 programs to 767 beds in 98 programs.

The shift to more community hospices is partly an economic one. Governments have not begun to fund palliative care programs in hospitals so some hospital programs that were pilot projects have had to close down. To meet some of the unmet needs of people who were dying, community groups began to visit patients and families in their homes and in hospitals. They raised money and awareness in the community about hospice care and incorporated themselves into community hospice groups. Many of these community groups began in smaller towns and cities where it is easier to get media attention and community funding.

Economic Analysis of Hospice Care

Adam Linton, former president of the Ontario Medical Association and a London, Ontario physician who died recently of cancer wrote a summary of what Ontario could do to improve health care and reduce costs. One of his conclusions was that the "public is constantly being told that much of medical care is not of proven value, and this is probably true."

Linton pointed out that many medical tests, treatments and operations are not proven effective but constantly performed. The Expert Panel on Palliative Care's Report to the Canadian Cancer Society's "Cancer 2000" task force estimated that "probably 75% of the total health care costs for a [patient's] life time" is spent in their last year of life. Were all the tests, treatments and surgeries necessary? Linton, and many others with similar experiences, would probably have said no. Too many people die in an intensive care unit (ICU) who should never have been there. They do not need high technological cures when they are dying. They need the compassionate and medically appropriate care for people who have a terminal or life-threatening illness. Dying is not a disease. Dying is the last stage of someone's life. People should be as pain free and alert as possible to enjoy this time, as best they can, with loved ones.

The *Report to Cancer 2000 Task Force by Expert Panel on Palliative Care* noted that the last year of life for a cancer patient in Canada is extremely expensive ("probably as much as 75% of the total health care costs for a [patient's] life time"). They concluded that even a slight shift in patterns of care for that last year of life would have great impact on costs for the health care system. These shifts would come through limiting relatively ineffective but expensive cancer therapies. "By questioning the goals of treatment, ensuring that the patient is giving informed consent, and by providing an active alternative approach in advanced disease, palliative care decreases costs. Governments and Cancer Centres must call into question treatment protocols that show minimal change in survival but add to the overall burden of suffering."

Later in their report the panel concludes that the "top priority for palliative care planning is to expand and upgrade palliative care services available in the home. This shift is partially in response to consumerism – people want to die in their own way and in their own space. However, the major motivation for this shift will be economic....In order to increase the proportion of advanced cancer patients living and dying in their home (perhaps up to 30-40%), we must find mechanisms and incentives to increase family participation. We should follow the lead of Scandinavian countries by reimbursing family members for lost income and expenses related to caring for cancer patients in the home." In the spirit of palliative care it would be natural to extend this recommendation to family members caring for those suffering from any type of terminal illness.

In a proposal submitted to the Ontario Provincial Government, Sunnybrook Health Science Centre together with the Whitelight Hospice Foundation prepared an analysis of hospice care versus general hospital care. The Foundation is a community initiative to establish a freestanding hospice for cancer patients in Metropolitan Toronto. Sunnybrook Health Science Centre is a major university teaching hospital in Metropolitan Toronto.

They argue that a lack of community alternatives for palliative care in the home means that hospitals must provide services to patients with a terminal illness. These patients take up beds intended for patients needing high technology tests, surgery, and treatments (acute care) to help cure their illness. To use hospital beds intended for acute care to provide palliative care is a misuse of health care dollars.

While home is the preferred location for much palliative care there are people who are unable to stay at home and need the services of either a free-standing hospice or a hospital. The Sunnybrook-Whitelight proposal estimates the savings of having a free-standing, 30-bed hospice facility with 85% occupancy the first year as follows:

Table 2.

Type of Bed	Cost Per Patient Day	Per Year
Acute Care Cancer Bed (average costs do not include doctor or operating room costs)	$600.00	$5,584,500
Hospice Bed	$273.79	$2,548,300
Cost Savings	$329.21	$3,036,200

This saving of $3,036,200 assumes that for each hospice bed there is a reduction in the number of cancer beds. Yet the increase in the number of registered cancer patients at the Toronto Bayview Regional Cancer Centre, also located on the campus of Sunnybrook Health Science Centre, has gone from 441 in 1980 to 4,251 in 1990 (almost ten times as many new cancer cases). It is unlikely, therefore, that cancer beds would be reduced by establishing a free-standing hospice. However, the hospice beds would provide the kind of services patients need while at the same time more patients asking for active cancer treatments would have acute care beds available for them.

According to many leaders in the field of hospice and health care, the most cost effective method of caring for people with a terminal illness is achieved by care provided to patients in their own homes. With a co-ordinated effort of home care, family support, community and/or hospital-based outreach programs, the cost for taking care of someone at home is substantially reduced especially since much of the work is done by family members, friends and/or volunteers. More specific data needs to be collected to support this claim. Hopefully, with the development of provincial and federal associations for palliative care there will be increased efforts to keep statistics on the number of patients and family members served, the costs for the different types of services and the physical, emotional, spiritual and informational benefits that such programs provide over those offered in traditional health care.

Wolf Wolfensberger, in his 1984 article, cautions us however about concentrating on costs, especially those paid for by governments. He says that in the United States federal funding regulations have perverted hospice programs in at least three ways. (a) Free-standing hospice services must be cheaper than hospital care. (b) Home care must cost less than free-standing hospice care. (c) Hospice services for people who are dying can only be funded for a very short period, e.g. six months. "The first two provisions are designed to protect and support the medical and nursing home economic empires. The third one imposes a tremendous dying role and expectancy upon the people served. Imagine accepting a hospice-for-the-dying service, and seeing your (six month) 'deadline' approaching! If you survive it, you feel almost obliged to apologize to all the people who fully expected you to die, and who now are saddled with all sorts of inconveniences and unpleasant obligations by the fact that you are hanging on or – God forbid – even recover." (p. 158)

Why We Spend So Much Money on Health Care

In 1987 Canadians spent about $47,935,000,000.00 on health care, or about 8.98% of the Gross National Product. That means that for every $100 of goods and services we produced in our country, $8.98 went to health care. Imagine the costs to individuals and families if they had to pay these costs themselves. In the U.S., for example, families paid an average of $1,742 per year for health care insurance in 1981. By 1990 that cost was on average $4,296. It is expected to increase to $9,397 by the year 2000 unless there are radical changes to health care funding in America.

When trying to understand modern health care costs in Canada we must understand that health care has become an industry rather than a charitable organization. Before World War II, Canada was a manufacturing, mining, forestry and farming country with health care often provided through religious and charitable organizations. Since the war, health care has become a major service industry in Canada and many people now depend on the health care system for their jobs. Until recently, health costs knew no limit and was almost totally funded by taxes, therefore, there was little accountability for costs or the benefits of various treatments. How can this be so? One reason is that modern health care, a previously natural phenomena, has become oriented towards medical emergencies requiring highly trained professionals and technological interventions. Consider the differences over the past 50 years in how we "treat" birth, aging and death. Once natural processes that happened at home, they are now often in-hospital events requiring medical intervention. We are one of the last countries in the world to recognize the value, for example, of midwives.

In fact many women can have babies without high technology interventions while still receiving pain relief if they choose. Many people who are dying do not need or request high-cost intensive care near the end of their lives. Aging is not a disease that requires people to be taken from their homes and put into nursing homes. In 1988-89 there were 5,101 residential facilities in Canada with 237,437 beds for people labelled with various diseases or disabilities, physical and mental. Of those institutions 2,239 were for "the aged" with 166,177 beds. In a survey of these institutions for older people 1,405 facilities reported that their total costs were $2,665,415,000 ($1,705,956,000 for staffing). Aging, itself, has become an industry in Canada unlike most every other country in the world including European countries and the U.S.

It is a national embarrassment that so much of our national income and employment comes from taking people out of their homes and putting them into institutions where trained professionals can "treat" people who do not know the alternative forms of care available in other countries. It is a national shame that must be changed for moral, as well as economic, reasons. People should not be taken from their homes to receive care (often unnecessary care). Whenever possible, people should be able to stay in their homes and have services brought to them. Palliative care, especially that provided at home, can help change how we help people who are dying and put some perspective back into how Canadians view dying and death as natural phenomena.

Politics of Palliative Care

The field of palliative care is young in Canada. Palliative care formally began here with the opening of the palliative care units in Winnipeg and Montreal in 1975. Since then the number and types of programs have increased as have the competition for funding and promoting one type of program over another.

There are some people who argue that good palliative care means good medical care. The assumption is that patients should receive all the physical, emotional, spiritual and informational supports they require through improved modern medical care. Others agree with this general argument but also believe that palliative care should be seen as a medical specialty and accorded special space and policies within a hospital to provide optimum care.

However, palliative care is not equal to good medical care, although perhaps it should be in the best of worlds. Palliative patients require the help of professional doctors and nurses, but, palliative care is more than physical or medical care. It is a philosophy of care that requires individual attention for every patient and family and is almost impossible to receive in a general hospital's treatment wards. Some people require greater support from medical and nursing staff while others require more support from family, friends, spiritual counsellors, social workers or various kinds of physio or occupational therapy. One model cannot provide all forms of palliative care regardless of the good intentions of the proponents of that model.

While leaders in the field discuss the importance of patient and family control over their lives, a real competition continues between programs for public support and funding. The philosophy of palliative care is sometimes lost to the daily administrative and political in-fighting within the field. To avoid this, more effort must be made to co-operate and co-ordinate the care given to patients and families. Patients and families are perceived as key members on a palliative care team yet many programs have no patient or family representation on their boards, standing committees or committees looking at standards of patient care. People with AIDS have clearly shown us that most people with a terminal or life-threatening illness have a real contribution to make in improving palliative care. They may one day receive palliative care and surely their perspective, concerns and needs must inform decision-making bodies.

The creation of provincial associations and the new Canadian Palliative Care Association are hopeful signs that the leaders within the field will bring together the various providers of care to improve the overall quality and numbers of programs available to Canadians across our nation.

If, however, the competition, especially between institutional and community hospice programs, is not addressed quickly then palliative care will remain a patchwork of programs that meet the needs of some individuals and families but will not be able to help enough of the more than 100,000 people who die of terminal or chronic illnesses every year. If palliative care providers do not begin to speak more with one voice in Canada then we will lose our power and credibility to affect changes in our health care and social services. If palliative care providers do not continue to respect and promote the various models of care, even at risk of losing some of their own plans, then people with a terminal illness will continue to die in general hospitals without the supports they need. If palliative care providers do not examine how programs can include people with heart, lung, and neuromuscular diseases then palliative care will become a philosophy and program limited only to people with cancer and perhaps AIDS. If palliative care providers do not begin to speak for women caregivers who have done most of the palliative care at home then these women will continue to struggle on without support and recognition. If palliative care providers do not begin to speak more for the children who are dying, for the children whose parents, grandparents or siblings have died, then these children will not receive the community and school supports they need. If palliative care providers do not expand the supports they provide each other, I fear we will lose those dedicated providers through exhaustion or frustration.

Many people in palliative care want to take leadership roles to build their ideal programs. There are no ideal programs and there will always be competing programs and services. All of us must begin to recognize the primary importance of the patient and family and the secondary importance of the programs and services. If not, I fear that palliative care will be folded into the traditional health and social services provided in Canada where administrative and bureaucratic considerations take precedence over people. Canadians have an opportunity to improve palliative care, and through this improvement, all health care if we work together with, and on behalf of, patients.

We need the various groups (patients, families, professionals, volunteers, policy makers and funders) involved in palliative care, health care and social services to meet to establish a long-term plan. They need to examine the universal palliative care options in the greater context of all health and social issues (e.g. poverty, housing, unemployment). They need to examine human and financial costs of proceeding, or not proceeding, with expanded and enhanced hospice care. They need to examine how health care and social service resources should be reallocated to meet the needs of all people who are dying and while also providing the supports needed by the families. They need to examine who does, and who should, be making health care decisions including treatment decisions made in the last year of someone's life. They need to examine alternatives to institutional care (i.e. hospitals, nursing homes, and other health care facilities) without just "dumping" people back into the community without adequate supports as happened in Ontario with deinstitutionalization of mental health facilities. They must examine how to educate professionals and the public alike about their rights and responsibilities in making health care decisions. They must examine the role of families (often women) who provide care at a great financial loss with inadequate support. This collective of people must do more than write another health care report. As a group they must demand and affect changes that will improve services and reduce mismanaged care.

What will happen if professional health caregivers' goals do not become secondary to a dying patient-family's goals? I fear that attention will continue to be drawn away from the issues of palliative care and move toward euthanasia as the solution to meeting the needs of people who are dying.

CHAPTER 5

STANDARDS OF CARE: HOW DO WE GET THE PALLIATIVE CARE WE NEED?

In 1991 I wrote an article for the December edition of the *Pain Management Newsletter* on palliative care standards. This chapter is based on that article and discusses the importance of standards in ensuring quality palliative care.

Standards are measuring tools to help professionals, volunteers, patients and families evaluate the type and quality of care they are giving or receiving. Standards are based on a clearly defined philosophy of palliative care. A palliative care program begins by defining its philosophy and goals and then writes out standards of care to put that philosophy into action. Standards can help palliative care programs improve their overall quality of service while making sure they remain true to their philosophy. Standards can, however, also restrict flexibility in providing care to individuals rather than to groups of patients. Thus the question of standards represents a challenge facing palliative care programs across Canada.

A discussion of standards is often as dry as one on a government budget but it is just as important. Canadians should understand how palliative care is designed, delivered and evaluated. Without broader participation of people within, and outside, of hospice care a small, elite group of people will determine what is the best kind of hospice care for the rest of us.

For people interested in palliative care it is important to understand how programs develop and how to evaluate their effectiveness. Philosophical statements, standards and policies and procedures will tell you a great deal about a specific program's approach to meeting the needs of individual people who have a terminal or life-threatening illness.

Palliative care standards are currently being designed by local and national organizations across Canada. These organizations generally lack significant input from patients, families, patient advocates, allied professionals and services, and community members.

Who Decides on the Design and Quality Assurance of Standards?

At present there are many groups and organizations discussing and developing palliative care standards. These groups include The Canadian Council on Health Facilities Accreditation (CCHFA); ministries of health, professional organizations (e.g. Ontario Medical Association), community hospices, hospital based palliative care programs, local/regional/provincial/national associations of palliative care providers and organizations (e.g. Canadian Palliative Care Association, Community Hospice Association of Ontario, Hospice Victoria, the British Columbia Palliative Care Association), advisory groups and individual programs.

Within this long list, however, there is little input from patients, families, patient advocates and the general community, nor is there much effort by many of these organizations to establish palliative care standards that reflect the differing alternatives of free standing hospices, community hospices (volunteer led), hospital-based palliative care programs, and regional palliative care services. There is also insufficient input from front-line allied professionals such as therapists, pharmacists and dieticians within palliative care and allied services such as home care, and other community services to ensure continuity of care.

Overview of Current Work:
The Components of Palliative Care Standards

Health and Welfare Canada's *Palliative-Care Services: Guidelines for Establishing Standards* sets out a functional classification of a palliative care program. This program design incorporates the components of administration, symptom control, psycho-social support, spiritual support, volunteers, bereavement support, program evaluation and training. Only the first four components are required for a clinical (medical) program. By definition these guidelines present a clinical model of palliative care. In using words such as "preliminary" to describe programs that do not have one of those four required components, the guidelines minimize the immense impact that many volunteer-based community hospice programs provide. There is the implication that such programs do not "measure up."

Furthermore, by insisting on such rigid standards, we may be excluding effective programs from future accreditation or licensing, which funders may require one day. Health care traditionally requires some form of accreditation for provincial funds. It will be standards that determine which programs will qualify. Therefore, we must be cautious about limiting the diversity and creativity of many programs that do not fit into a more traditional medical model of care.

Certainly we need standards of patient care. However, this does not mean that groups of health care professionals alone should determine what constitutes a palliative care program. Program standards can limit a vital element of the palliative care philosophy, namely, providing a flexible and adaptable level of care depending on the client's (patient and family) expressed needs. From a client's perspective, a community hospice program of volunteers working together with a family physician, homecare and the hospice's own nursing staff might be the best possible program. By limiting the options, a rigid set of standards could in effect deny a person the sort of program best suited to his or her situation. The fact is, one program is not inherently better than the other. There are different programs because there are different people with different needs.

Choosing the Major Components

How then do programs choose the major components of care within their standards? There are at least two systems available. The first is a synthesis of the standards work already done by such groups as the CCHFA (Canadian Council on Health Facilities Accreditation) coupled with specific research presented in the literature. There is already substantial consensus on these peer evaluation standards. [Note: accreditation councils establish standards based on review of organized health delivery by professional peers rather than consumer evaluation.] The second is a client-centred and client-evaluated system.

The CCHFA 1990 standards provide an approach in which the emphasis is on organization, policies and procedures but the core standards still emphasize patient care components. The standards are: (1) statement of purpose, goals and objectives; (2) organization and direction; (3) policies and procedures developed by staff, management & internal and external services and communicated to patients and families; (4) human and physical resources; (5) orientation, staff development and continuing education; (6) patient care; and (7) quality assurance.

The advantage of using the CCHFA standards is that these standards must be adhered to by 1992 in all accredited health care facilities across Canada. Therefore some consistency of program and professional skills evaluation between institutional and community programs would be provided.

The second system is a client-centred evaluation system. Wolfensberger has designed an evaluation process in social services that could be adapted to the field of palliative care. Among other components, his methods measure degree of individual /client control, the degree to which program and staff encourage client self-determination, the importance of physical location and layout of services, the use of signs and symbols, continuity of care, the human aspects of care, confidentiality, and advocacy.

However it is achieved, I recommend that any palliative care standards should be a combination of a peer evaluation and client evaluated system of standards and quality assurance.

Questions to Consider

The following is a list of concerns/questions that might be addressed before any group finalizes its palliative care standards and quality assurance programs.

Recognize the individual and group values and how they are reflected in the standards. Will those values incorporate the beliefs and needs of clients who have different cultures, languages, educational backgrounds, economic abilities, religions, sexual orientations, and personal histories? Do the values incorporate people who have diseases other than cancer? Is the group primarily a white, middle/upper class, educated, English/French speaking one? If yes, how can the program encourage greater diversity of representation in staff, clients and volunteers to reach a wider community?

Do the standards reflect a program approach, a discipline approach or a client-centred approach? A program approach (similar to the "Palliative Care Services Guidelines") emphasizes the interdisciplinary aspects of palliative care. The discipline approach defines the professional and clinical standards for each discipline (medicine, nursing, chaplaincy, etc.) similar to acute care settings today. A client-centred approach would concentrate on the palliative care philosophy of having the patient and family as the central component to any program or its evaluation.

Are patients and families involved in helping design and evaluate standards? If yes, are they involved to the same degree as other members of the palliative care team? If not, why not? People with cancer, heart disease, AIDS, neuromuscular diseases, and others are all capable of discussing their needs and wants (indeed, they already do some of this through support groups, with palliative care teams, with the media, and with their families).

Do the standards imply that dying is a disease or illness or, more appropriately, do the standards imply that people are going through a final process of living?

Do the standards incorporate a quality assurance program that meets both the client and staff needs? A general rule of QA is that you get what you inspect more often than what you expect. Standards do not ensure behavioral and attitudinal changes without effective senior management, a sound philosophy (mission statement), and role modelling of expected behaviours.

Do the standards include what quality assurance experts call RUMBA measurements to evaluate standards? RUMBA represents measurements that are *relevant*, *understandable* to clients and staff, *measurable* (quantifiable), *behavioral* and *achievable* over time and under predictable circumstances.

Are interpersonal skills clearly defined in the standards, for example: ensuring privacy, confidentiality, informed choices, concern, empathy, honesty, tact, and sensitivity to meet the individual, social and technical performance expectations?

Is palliative care clearly defined in the mission statement and goals? Does the program include only people who have a life expectancy of less than six months or does it assume that palliative care begins with the onset of illness?

Do the standards recognize that people die as they have lived and that families react to a loved one's dying as they react to other major stressors? (Therefore, patients and families will not want to behave in accordance with standards that run counter to their traditional ways of living.)

Do the standards recognize that no one will die "perfectly" regardless of what the standards are? When we offer choices, people will not always choose what professionals think is in their best interest. Standards should allow for that flexibility and sensitivity to client and family needs.

Further Considerations

We will all be patients one day unless we die very suddenly. We must recognize the invaluable contribution that clients, frontline staff and volunteers have to make in designing and evaluating palliative care standards. Many other industries (and remember that health care is an industry) recognize the role of "customer satisfaction" in designing, implementing and evaluating their services.

We should use this historical opportunity to set the future trends for health care in Canada. In the United States many hospice programs are bogged down in funding formulas, administrative headaches and management issues. Critics suggest that many have forgotten their original mission and have mirrored the difficulties faced by acute care facilities.

There is competition between palliative care programs for money and political recognition. Professionals within the field must cooperate in their efforts to improve palliative care in Canada. Professionals must establish concurrent client-centred standards to balance the peer evaluation standards that are being designed at present. We should develop, over time, an independent method of evaluating programs that incorporate a client-centred approach similar to Wolfensberger's approach. This independent method would supplement the peer evaluation methods of groups such as the CCHFA.

Patients and families must understand both their rights and their responsibilities for working together with professionals and volunteers to provide the best care possible. Patients play an active role in taking care of themselves as do their families, yet we often only evaluate the professionals and volunteers in our programs.

CHAPTER 6

REFLECTIONS ON PALLIATIVE CARE: VOICES FROM THE FRONT LINE

The thoughts, ideas and concerns of Canadian leaders in this field are especially important at this time in Canada hospice care, as provincial and national associations and governments begin to develop longer-term plans.

Although this chapter highlights the thoughts of some palliative care experts there is a whole group of people not represented – patients and families. I do not often work directly with patients and families so I have no consistent access to people who receive palliative care services and those who do not. At some point I hope that this expert group of patients and families will have their thoughts, beliefs and hopes recorded for public debate as well (perhaps in a future edition of this book).

Modern palliative care began in the late 1960s in England with the work of Dame Cicely Saunders and her St. Christopher's Hospice. It began in Canada in 1975 with the opening of a two palliative care units; one in St. Boniface Hospital in Winnipeg and the other at the Royal Victoria Hospital in Montreal.

What has been accomplished in Canada in 17 years? I asked palliative care experts, both professional and volunteer, to summarize some of the major successes of Canadian palliative care. What follows is an overview of their responses. I have tried to quote comments that represent the views of a number of these leaders to show the broad outlines of agreement and disagreement.

Pain and Symptom Control

Most of the palliative leaders recognized the immense improvements in pain management especially for people who have cancer. Dr. Balfour Mount, the physician who was instrumental in opening up the palliative care unit at the Royal Victoria Hospital listed "improved pain control" as the first success of palliative care in Canada. Keep in mind, however, that since fewer than five percent of Canadians receive services from palliative care programs, there is still a long way to go. The skills and techniques are available now to provide effective pain and symptom control if only enough physicians acquired and practised these techniques. There are physicians practicing effective pain management in Canada without working through a palliative care program but these skilled physicians still remain in the minority.

Dr. Dorothy Ley, the founder and past president of the Palliative Care Foundation adds that "we are better at understanding pain and managing it. We are not perfect. There are lots of doctors that still deny the basic tenets of pain management. Young doctors appear more interested in the principles of pain management and some are even interested in the broader philosophy of palliative care."

Volunteer Initiative and Community Hospices

Another success mentioned by many of the leaders in the field was the initiative shown by community volunteers in developing and maintaining community hospice and hospital palliative care programs. Heather Balfour, Executive Director of the Community Hospice Association of Ontario says the "reliance on volunteers by many community-based hospices has meant the grassroots development of a cost-efficient and dedicated human resource for hospice/palliative care." Catherine A. Rakchaev, Executive Director of the Dorothy Ley Hospice, points out that hospices emerged from the grass roots level in many cases. Without the volunteers many of these programs would never have started. These volunteers include health care professionals: people working in health care who helped create programs that were not present in their own settings. Dr. Margaret Scott, Associate Professor of Medicine and Provincial Palliative Care Consultant in Newfoundland adds that "many community-based programs are giving excellent care."

Patient-Family Awareness and Rights

Trinity Hospice Toronto members summarize community hospice programs as "client focused where the client is in control, the family and client are cared for as one unit with mutual supports, team efforts and community involvement."

Gertrude Paul, a Palliative Care Consult Nurse in Brockville, says that "a greater public awareness of dying with dignity in institutions and at home" is a success of hospice care. Her colleague, Barbara Noonan, confirms that "palliative care has made death and dying more an approachable subject and made people aware of their rights." A lawyer with specific expertise in palliative care (who prefers anonymity) states: "the greatest success is the increased public awareness of a patient's right to choose a course of treatment and, if necessary, to reject certain courses of treatments. However, this is an ongoing process and greater efforts to educate the public are required."

Marilynne Seguin, Executive Director of Dying with Dignity and a nurse herself, believes "the introduction of palliative care and hospice services in Canada have greatly improved the options for the terminally ill in Canada. Dying With Dignity unreservedly supports both the trend and the movement. At the same time we cannot lose sight of the fact that the choice of care is the prerogative of a person who is making decisions about the end of their life. For some persons the services provided either by a palliative care team or through hospice is the very best alternative for their personal situation."

Wilma O'Connell, also a Coordinator of Palliative Care (Brockville) summarized this point. A major accomplishment in Canadian palliative care is, "improved communication and acceptance that the patient has the right to accept or refuse treatment and should be supported in their choice."

Development of Programs

Palliative care may have started in many different ways across Canada but as Wilma O'Connell explains with such enthusiasm: "Palliative care is a reality in our health care system! It does enhance the quality of life for our patients and families. The terminally ill have the right to be heard and cared for by professionals and volunteers who believe it is a privilege to support the dying." Her colleague Cheryl Chapman (a Community Outreach Coordinator) says that more people see "palliative care as the norm versus the exception."

Larry Grossman, Physician Manager of the Palliative Care Unit at Scarborough Grace Hospital, notes as another success the "development of both hospital-based and community-based programs in spite of lack of funding. The involvement of ALL members of health care team in patient care and planning is a further success." Perhaps this interdisciplinary model will be translated to other areas of health care as well. Dr. Dorothy Ley agrees that "professionals in the various field are beginning to work more together in teams. There is also growing medical and nursing acceptance of the other allied professionals (e.g. social workers, chaplains, therapists) as part of the support team helping patients." Dr. Balfour Mount reminds us of some of our "models of care that have been copied elsewhere" indicating the excellence these programs have achieved.

Professor Tom Malcomson of George Brown College in Toronto, who teaches issues of dying and death, sees one of the key areas of success in palliative care as the "many different groups and networks established to provide palliative care. The fact there is no systemization of the whole range is good. Hopefully, they will remain fractured and providing different programs" [to meet the individual needs of people who are dying rather than fulfilling bureaucratic criteria of services].

Palliative Care Units for Teaching Professional Caregivers

Dr. Margaret Scott stressed "the establishment of teaching units at Montreal, Winnipeg, Edmonton, Quebec City, Ottawa, Halifax, Vancouver and Newfoundland" as major successes. She believes another success is the "medical school recognition of education needs with specific examples of the Universities of Edmonton, Toronto, McMaster, Ottawa, Dalhousie and Memorial University in Newfoundland."

Cost Effectiveness of Community Palliative Care Programs

Jackie MacKenzie, Executive Director of Hospice of London, believes that community hospices are "a cost effective outreach to a great number of clients and a positive benefit to families. Their emphasis on health promotion for family caregivers at home is invaluable."

Palliative Care Associations and Conferences

Several of the palliative care leaders mentioned as successes the development of palliative care associations and conferences. Shirley Cooper, a bereavement counsellor in Brockville, believes that "Canadian palliative care's greatest successes are the development of provincial organizations and also the yearly Canadian Conferences and International Conferences" held every two years in Montreal. Dr. Larry Grossman believes these organizations "have taken the lead in education, guidelines to be followed, standards to be aimed at etc." in the improvement of palliative care services across Canada. Dr. Balfour Mount is justifiably proud of the Montreal International Congress which he has spearheaded as "a forum for exchange of information and a catalyst for growth" with people coming from around the world to attend.

The Human and Spiritual Successes

The Reverend Sally Eaton, Chaplain at Toronto's The Wellesley Hospital, sees an "increased public awareness of death, the grief process, and a beginning to see death as part of life again." Dr. Larry Grossman sees a "broadening of vision from pain and symptom control to a more holistic approach to patients."

Dr. Dorothy Ley believes that the general public and professionals alike are more aware of the needs of people who are dying. "I know there is a growing feeling that you can die at home. It's tough and difficult and is not always possible but it is more acceptable then 15 years ago. There is a growing acknowledgement of the spiritual nature of dying and illness and I think palliative care has done that. The importance of the chaplain is finally being recognized."

Steven Waring, a hospice volunteer with Hospice Dufferin in Orangeville, Ontario, believes that hospice brings "an awareness to the community – society – of the needs of the dying person, the family and the bereavement process. Hospice can bring humanity to an often fearful experience."

Bridging Past Successes to Future Development

Dr. Elizabeth Latimer, Director of Palliative Care, Hamilton Civic Hospitals, sees palliative care "as being in the early to middle stages of developing. We are more aware – now we need to ask questions: (1) Where have we come from?, (2) What do we have?, and (3) How many (what %) of people in need are being served?"

This chapter has answered part of her first question. Chapter 4 identified some of what we have now by way of palliative care programs in Canada. The answer to her third question requires national, provincial and local coordination of data collection to get a real picture of how many people, patients and family members, are being served out of the total population that would like these services.

Summary of Successes

- improved pain and symptom control techniques (although not understood and practised by enough doctors)
- initiative of grass roots to begin hospice programs
- early concentration on the palliative care philosophy of patient-family centred care
- increased public awareness of palliative care (still a long way to go) and increased discussions on issues of dying and death
- increased understanding of patient's right to accept and refuse treatments
- increased acceptance of palliative care as part of the continuum of health care with a multi-disciplinary approach to care
- increased acceptance of palliative care in hospitals, in patients' homes and in free-standing hospices
- increased number and quality of palliative care conferences and workshops for professionals and volunteers
- increased cooperation between professionals, volunteers and provincial-national associations.

Where do we want to be in the year 2000? The next chapter looks at some of the personal visions people have for Canadian palliative care at the turn of the century.

CHAPTER 7

PALLIATIVE CARE IN THE YEAR 2000: WHAT WE NEED TO DO

What should Canadian palliative care look like in the year 2000? What needs to happen to get us there? Again I turned to the leaders in the field.

Variety of Choices for Patients

Most responses regarding hopes for palliative care spoke of the provision of a wide range of program choices for people who are dying. This range of programs includes informal home-based support teams, community hospices, and hospital-based programs.

Professor Tom Malcomson who teaches on issues of dying and death wrote "If someone I loved was dying, I would want to take care of them in the home (theirs, mine or ours). I would want to be able to provide pain medication, know the contraindications, know the side effects, provide proper bed care and nutrition. Friends, neighbours and family would help in the care of the dying person. Money would be available to help defray costs and lost income while I cared for my loved person. It would not entail a system of health care professionals taking the responsibility and human contact away and assuming responsibility for the dying person. It would be difficult, painful and troubling (feelings of every mix would be present), but it would be a more natural, human, connected death for the other person and myself."

Carol Derbyshire, Executive Director of Hospice of Windsor, is "a firm believer that the back bone of a good palliative care program is the volunteer component. Volunteers who are carefully screened and well trained and monitored are a tremendous asset to the organization. On the other hand, I feel that it is important to have paid staff also because someone must be accountable at all times. Staff should also be well screened and trained. This area of work draws many 'needy' people. We all need to be needed but a balance must be maintained. Often times staff forget whose needs we are here to meet. This can be disastrous if not identified."

Shirley Cooper, a Bereavement Coordinator, states her "personal vision of palliative care for the 21st century as home-based [programs] complimented with a staff of visiting nurses for personal care and other professionals to help deal with the psychosocial and grief aspects. Hospitalization should be available, however, for respite, chemotherapy, and monitoring pain."

The Reverend Sally Eaton wants to see hospice care "available to all, with more free-standing hospices, teams in all major hospitals and/or dedicated hospice beds. In smaller communities I would like to see volunteer and/or paid teams that crossover between community and hospital and have more volunteer teams like All Saint's Hospice (Ottawa) and Trinity Hospice Toronto to augment in-home family care."

Dr. Larry Grossman would like to see hospice care "integrated into primary practice or community health care – institutional care should be a safety net, not a catchall. We need much better coordination and communication between hospitals, primary care doctors and community services. New programs should all have an outreach component. Need better access to beds for emergency admissions and resources for 'crisis' intervention in the home."

Evelyn MacKay, former nurse, therapeutic touch practitioner and palliative care volunteer and teacher, agrees with Dr. Grossman. In her vision hospice care is "away from the seduction of high tech hospital units! People should be dying at home but with such trips to small palliative care units as are necessary to maintain comfort. Increase teams of educated caregivers (such as Victorian Order of Nurses), increase supplies for physical illnesses – so we must expand the provincial homecare programs. Free-standing hospices are isolationist and tough for staff." This last comment is in contradiction to, for example, Reverend Sally Eaton's comment above.

Steven Waring, a community hospice volunteer notes, hospice care should be "providing excellence in trust, pain control, comfort and humanity for the dying person and family as a unit of care. It should be totally available and accessible on a community basis. We should be shaping society's attitudes towards death and the whole of life – the community of life-caring for dying persons as part of society."

Jackie MacKenzie adds that along with improved co-ordination of programs without duplication of services must come "more family support to encourage caregiving at home and discourage fear, anxiety and exhaustion which often culminates in frustrating and costly admissions to institutions."

Dr. Dorothy Ley believes that palliative care units should be available only in teaching hospitals so they can be used for research and teaching the body of knowledge of palliative care to other professionals. In other hospitals, palliative care teams should be used to instruct hospital staff how to provide good palliative care including spiritual care, counselling, excellent hospice medical and nursing care.

Members of Wellington Hospice in Guelph, Ontario want to see the "widespread application of the hospice concept based largely on a volunteer basis. Free-standing hospices should be in each community."

Funding Issues

There is disagreement around the issue of who should fund hospice care. Many people would like to see palliative care receive full government funding while others prefer mixed funding sources (i.e. government and community fundraising) so that no single funder can regulate or dictate the kinds of palliative care a group provides.

Doctors Larry Grossman and Balfour Mount agree that adequate funding for palliative care beds should be provided to meet the needs of a growing population as part of the continuum of medical care provided in hospitals. Catherine A. Rakchaev believes that we need a coordinated, integrated, multidisciplinary service which is funded and marketed with services available in longterm care and acute care facilities, free-standing hospices and home supports. Education in all those facilities and in the community is required.

Cheryl Chapman writes "It's time this field of expertise was acknowledge as a bona fide necessary service – too much time is 'wasted' by service providers raising money when time and effort could go to direct patient care."

Laurie Bennett, Executive Director of Hospice of Peel has concerns about government funding however. "While I'm aware that most people who are involved in community-based hospices want and are lobbying for funding from the provincial government, I have some serious reservations and concerns about going this route for funding. I feel that there is a real danger if community-based hospices were to receive either core funding or more than about 20% of their needed revenues from government because we could quite easily lose our autonomy and very quickly fall into the bureaucratic model, red tape, paperwork and rigid eligibility criteria of most government institutions. There is also the danger that the cost of community-based hospice services would increase simply because more money was available. Because most hospices don't receive government funding at present, we are forced to provide our services within the budgets of the money we are able to raise ourselves. Good quality and much needed services are being provided by community-based hospices now without government funding in most cases. Do we really need a lot more money and would more money (i.e. government funding) mean more and better hospices services?"

A separate funding issue is the way that physicians are paid for providing services. Most physicians in Canada are still paid on a "fee for service" basis. This means that they receive a set fee for every service they provide. Such a fee structure encourages physicians to provide as many services as possible within a day for them to earn the best income possible. In palliative care where one of the greatest skills required is time spent communicating with patients, the fee-for-service system does not work. Time spent visiting patients in their homes and spending an hour or so going through the various choices that patients have is not paid well by the fee-for-service system. Dr. Dorothy Ley believes that if we want physicians to spend time with us and to provide excellent palliative care supports to us, then they must be compensated for their time, expertise and transportation costs. Physicians who provide palliative care support in people's homes are presently penalized with much lower incomes than their colleagues and they provide this service at a cost to their personal and family lives as well since palliative care is not easily practised during regular business hours.

Education

Education is seen as a key factor in the hospice care of the year 2000. Dr.

Balfour Mount would like to see academic programs in all Canadian medical schools with Canadian multi-centre clinical trials held for research and teaching purposes. Dr. Margaret Scott would like to see physicians taught palliative care as part of "the full medical care of all 'end stage' patients." Doctors need to acquire a "full awareness of therapeutic options" available to them to help patients who are dying.

Dr. Elizabeth Latimer's views on palliative care education include the "need to work with patients and families but we must also try to do the more difficult tasks of (1) educating colleagues, (2) public education, (3) dissemination of information. These tasks will not always be popular with health professionals because they need to learn and change, but I believe that most patients will be best served if more and more practitioners can become committed to palliative care and educated about it."

Heather Balfour says "I believe the established and new palliative care programs are suffering from a lack of public recognition. The general public needs to be educated as to what hospice/palliative care is and needs to create a lobby for adequate resources to provide palliative care."

Dr. Balfour Mount agrees that there must be increased pressure on our political representatives, along with increased public grassroots demand, to ensure the proper place of palliative care in meeting the needs of people with a terminal or life-threatening illness.

Dr. Louis Dionne, Director General of Maison Michel Sarrazin (Sillery, Quebec), summarizes his views in concise language "Teach. . . Teach. . . Teach." Through focusing on provincial palliative care associations, involving the community, and through teaching professionals and volunteer groups we can "promote palliative care to the society."

Broadening the Scope of Palliative Care

Dr. Dorothy Ley wants palliative care to broaden its base, regardless of the disease. The palliative care philosophy of care should be available to people regardless what their illness is. It must be available when someone's illness is not curable but when we can, and should, provide active, compassionate care so we can stop the "there is nothing more we can do" attitude in health care.

Virginia Clark Weir, Manager of Continuing and Palliative Care at Scarborough Grace Hospital believes that at present "palliation is associated with cancer for the most part – many patients suffering from long-term illnesses other than cancer would greatly benefit from a more universal palliation approach. There is a need to work to allay the FEAR of health care workers in dealing with patients suffering chronic and end stage disease and impending death. Best way to allay these fears is often to communicate by example."

Jackie MacKenzie wants people to receive care earlier on in their illness as well. "Supportive care should be provided at the time of life-threatening diagnosis. This support could be through individual and group teaching and support sessions, with a consistent support present as client and family approach death and ultimately bereavement. Key here is empowering people to make decisions appropriate to them based on correct information. I see more clients wishing to remain at home with institutions or free-standing hospices meeting client or family emergencies only."

Through earlier referral to palliative care programs (e.g. at time of diagnosis of a terminal illness) Marilynne Seguin believes that another broader role for palliative care is that of acting as a patient advocate. The role of advocate "is not to sway [a patient's] decision in any one direction, but rather to assist the patient, the family and health care providers in examining all alternatives and then to support the patient in their choice of care. . . . The role of the advocate: (1) to ensure the person is fully informed of their diagnosis and prognosis; (2) ensure they understand as fully as possible the implications of the same on physical, emotional, social, financial and spiritual aspects of their life; (3) explore all alternative decisions that could be made; (4) when the person has reached their decision, to work toward resolution; and (5) seek healing within the family in dealing with the death."

Standards of Care

Many people within the field of palliative care want to see regional, provincial and/or national standards of professional and volunteer care provided to people with a terminal or life-threatening illness. From standards would come evaluations of services provided to patients and families and this quality assurance would finally provide a statistical analysis of what Canadian hospice care is doing well and not so well.

Dr. Dorothy Ley believes that along with peer review standards of care (see Chapter 5) there must also be clinical standards set for physicians, nurses, social workers, chaplains, etc. to ensure that the highest quality of professional care is taught, provided and evaluated.

Physician standards of clinical practice, for example, would include what knowledge and expertise they would need to have to help patients who are dying. The standards would describe expectations of physicians to provide satisfactory pain and symptom control. The standards might describe the expectations of a physician's role in a multi-disciplinary approach to health care in general, and within the specific area of palliative care.

Spiritual Concerns

Many people within palliative care recognize the immense value of a patient and family's sense of spirituality. No where else in our medical system is the spiritual element so readily accepted as in palliative care.

The Reverend Sally Eaton believes we must go farther with the spiritual elements of palliative care. There is a "great need to give the spiritual care component the place it deserves alongside psychosocial, physical, emotional components of patient/family care. By this I do not mean having a pastor or prayer book handy; rather that all disciplines ought to be trained to recognize the spiritual dimension and refer to a professional when appropriate. Spiritual questions have to do with questions of meaning, the purpose of life, the BIG questions that we ignore until they hit us in the face in a time of crisis. They are universal, and relatively few people today have religious ways of dealing with these questions."

Dr. Dorothy Ley adds the dimension of gratitude in her presentations on the importance of spirituality in palliative care. She believes that some people need help in understanding their new limitations and help in looking at all they have to be grateful about in their present situation rather than lamenting what they no longer can do. This journey of recognizing the happiness and love evident at a time when someone is very ill is spiritual and powerful in helping people identify the meaning of their own past and the meaning of their life at present.

Helping others identify what they have to be grateful for now also helps caregivers identify what they have in their lives that deserve their gratitude. Few people work in palliative care who do not examine their own lives in a new light of what is important and what is not as important as they once thought. Professionals and volunteers alike in palliative care often change their life goals and priorities and try to spend more of their time and efforts at improving communication with their own loved ones.

However, people in palliative care do not always take the necessary time to look at how they can support each other. Many palliative care programs have team meetings and sessions to discuss their thoughts, concerns, feelings of loss when someone dies. This is one reason why the turnover in professional staff is so low in palliative care. However, people who spend most of their time caring for other people sometimes forget to take care of themselves.

Cheryl Chapman sums up the need for caregivers to take better care of themselves and each other in this way. "Support one another – be gentle with each other and ourselves. We can't keep going on without human compassion for each other. I have talked with many palliative care support personnel from Europe, U.S.A., Canada, Australia, New Zealand, Britain, and a lack of support is prevalent internationally, not just in 'your hospital' or 'your province'. Remember why we are in this work – for the patient and family – and therefore when experiencing 'territorial' behaviour amongst colleagues, think of who is getting lost in the argument – the patient and family. Work as a team, respect roles of everyone, acknowledge work well done, give the pats on the back and songs of praise!"

The Human Dimension

Palliative care is about caring for people who have a terminal or life-threatening illness and caring for their family. As we saw above, good palliative care also means that professionals and volunteers take care of themselves and each other. Joanne C. Oosterhuis-Giliam, Clinical Director, Hopewell Children's Homes in Ontario, believes that true palliative care comes from the concept of "do not join, become." The palliative care movement is not about joining a new 'cause' but becoming a part of a philosophy of living the reflects and role models our commitment to other human beings through the palliative care philosophy of physical, emotional, spiritual and information supports for people who are dying.

Dr. Dorothy Ley believes this comes through professionals and volunteers learning to observe the people they are helping, getting to know them personally as people first, learning to communicate in ways that the person understands, and understanding that each of us as individuals cannot do it all – we need the help, support and practical skills of other professionals and volunteers. Palliative care requires people who care about others.

When provided well, Dr. Ley further believes, palliative care also means that as few different people as possible are involved in that care. At present someone living at home until their death may have more than 20 people coming from homecare, visiting home nurses, community hospice groups, etc. One homecare service may send out five different nurses to see the same patient in one week rather than consistently sending the same nurse who can build a rapport with the patient. Dr. Ley contends strongly that these scheduling issues must be addressed so that a minimum number of consistent caregivers can provide true hospice care at home or in a hospital.

The Reverend Sally Eaton suggests that "part of a vision [for palliative care in the year 2000] would be to have death and grief 'out of the closet' in our society and this can only come as fear of death, dying and illness is reduced." This reduction of fear can come about through what Dr. Larry Grossman calls "REACHING OUT – people with terminal illnesses are still alive, still have feelings, still have desires, still have goals, etc. Often patients and families feel shunned, or are reluctant to ask for support because of a fear of being treated like lepers. We need to recognize and capitalize on people's strengths and previous patterns of behaviour – relationships, hobbies, humour, etc. Need to provide an environment of caring and celebration, not distance and depression."

Professor Wolf Wolfensberger, Professor of Special Education at Syracuse University and developer of a client-centred evaluation tool of Human Service programs, summarizes the human dimension of palliative care. "We must distinguish between programs that respond to the specific needs of patients and family versus programs that respond to the needs of policies and procedures, laws, funding formulas, and professional pressures for conformity." In his view, only programs that provide true client-centred support can come close to simulating the ideal situation of a person living at home with the informal supports of family, friends, neighbours, and community resources (including the family physician) thereby avoiding the need for intrusive or paternalistic health care.

In his 1984 article he describes what he feels is an appropriate service for people who are dying. "Such a service also needs to be based on a positive ideology that does not succumb to any of the extremes of death denial, death obsession, or death glorification. Fortunately, we have some models. Some families have assumed the care of dying persons with minimal outside help, and some communal bodies have cared for their dying members – sometimes for years. Further, there are seven homes for poor dying people in the United States operated by the Hawthorne Dominican Servants without any subsidies from government or charge to patients or families. In fact, St. Christopher's in London was partially modeled on them in the first place." (p. 158)

Summary of Needs

- provide a wide range of program choices to everyone who wants/needs it
- increased information to patients and families of what they can do and what they can expect
- increase the volunteer component
- increase home care supports to patients and families with hospital back-ups for pain and symptom control
- increase teaching of professionals in university teaching hospitals through professional conferences and workshops
- increase co-ordination of programs
- address funding needs
- increase awareness and education of patients, families and the community in general
- broaden base of patients who are served by palliative care to
- include people who have illnesses other than cancer or AIDS
- refer patients earlier to palliative care programs so that they receive the physical, emotional, spiritual and informational supports when they need them most
- incorporate role of patient advocate to help patients understand their various options
- decide on the types and standards of care

- increase understanding of the spiritual component of care
- increase the amount of emotional supports provided to professional and volunteer caregivers
- increase patient-centred care.

CHAPTER 8

EUTHANASIA: COMMON ARGUMENTS FOR AND AGAINST

Whether or not to legalize euthanasia is, I believe, the wrong question. As I stated in the Introduction to this book, I believe that concentration on the narrow euthanasia debate detracts energy, resources and funding from developing and enhancing hospice care. In my opinion, a request for euthanasia is primarily a response to health care and social service systems that do not meet the needs of most people who are dying. At the same time I believe people do need an overview of the euthanasia debate to help them clarify their own thoughts.

When *Choices* was first published in 1986 I received many comments about the book and its objective presentation on the choices available to people who had a terminal or life-threatening illness. One of the most encouraging comments was about the chapter on euthanasia and its unemotional presentation of both sides of the debate. Most of that chapter appears below as an overview of the euthanasia debate.

Euthanasia, like abortion, capital punishment, war, suicide, and medical experimentation, is a very contentious and emotional issue. People who hold strong feelings either for or against euthanasia will not change their opinions based on anything in this chapter. If, however, people with strong views for or against euthanasia can read this chapter and find arguments to support their beliefs, then I have succeeded in presenting the issues fairly. If people who are undecided can find this information useful in helping them make up their mind then my purpose will be achieved.

Euthanasia stems from the Greek words *eu* (well) and *thanatos* (death). It refers to a painless and happy death. In modern usage it generally refers to the deliberate ending of someone else's life, with or without their consent, for compassionate reasons, when people are termi-nally ill or their suffering has become unbearable. Proponents of eu-thanasia argue that because of modern medical technology, it has be-come very difficult to die a natural death. The majority of North Ameri-cans die in hospitals where it is increasingly difficult to die as a direct result of a disease. Medical intervention, it is argued, prolongs death unnecessarily.

Two Types of Euthanasia

Euthanasia has often been broken up into two main divisions:

1. Active euthanasia involves someone, other than the persons who have a terminal, chronic or life-threatening illness, deliberately killing those persons (with or without their voluntary consent) by giving them a lethal dose of drugs, or ending their perceived suffering in any other direct way. Euthanasia by such violent acts as shooting or strangulation are considered "mercy killing" and are not seen as appropriate forms of killing by most people who approve of active euthanasia.

2. The right to refuse treatments (also called passive euthanasia by some) is legal in Canada in many situations. It involves someone, other than the person dying, allowing that person, with or without their volun-tary consent, not to begin or continue life-sustaining treatment. These life-sustaining treatments may include life-support machines, artificial feedings or hydration, or active treatments aimed at curing a disease. For example Jehovah Witnesses have the legal right in Canada to refuse blood transfusions that may save their lives.

The right to refuse treatment has been referred to as euthanasia by omission while active euthanasia is euthanasia by commission of a direct action. Often, the right to refuse treatment is requested directly by the person dying, either verbally or through a written document such as a 'living will'.

The right to refuse treatment, when voluntarily requested by a pa-tient, grants patients legal autonomy over medical decisions related to their care. The patient's legal rights blur, however, when health care-givers, family members or community members question a patient's mental competence to make these decisions. The legal questions be-come even more difficult when a patient is in some form of a coma, in a permanent vegetative state or experiencing dementia.

The argument against the distinction between right to refuse treatment and active euthanasia is that, whether you directly or indirectly cause someone's death, your intention and the resulting death are the same. Some argue that a doctor who allows a patient to refuse intravenous feedings, medications, surgery or a resuscitator, gets the same result as a doctor who gives a lethal dose of medication. This ethical and legal debate about whether or not active and passive euthanasia are morally indistinguishable will not be resolved quickly.

Reasons Some People Want Euthanasia

Euthanasia on the grounds of intractable or unbearable pain is becoming less of an issue. Pain control techniques are so effective that over 90 percent of people can be pain free and mentally alert until shortly before their death. However, many patients still suffer needless pain because of inadequate pain management by their doctors. The more pain control techniques are understood by doctors, the less the cry for euthanasia. For people who still have unbearable pain, medications can be given to put the person in a drug-induced coma to relieve physical suffering. If the person remains alive for some time they are brought out of the coma every few days to see if the pain is better controlled and they can return to being more alert.

The early 20th century American feminist Carrie Chapman Catt wrote that "no grief, pain, misfortune or 'broken heart' is an excuse for cutting off one's life while any power of service remains." She committed suicide during the terminal stages of her cancer after she decided she could no longer serve.

The argument for a quality of life is very important to those who support euthanasia. The basis of this argument is that individuals have the right to decide when their lives no longer have a quality that they want to live with. Defining "quality of life" is very difficult and it is unique to each individual. One person who is terminally ill, bedridden, and dependent on others will choose to live as fully as possible while someone else may ask to die.

Examining someone's quality of life can serve another purpose, however. If we know that some people are uncomfortable with their quality of life we can determine in what areas their lives can be improved or supported through such services as hospice care, increased visits by family and friends, and a continuing environment of support that shows the person they are valued members of their community. Using a numerical scale to define quality of life, however, is extremely dangerous and may well lead to even more premature deaths.

A last consideration for people who may choose euthanasia is financial. People who are dying worry a great deal about their families. They do not want to be an emotional burden, nor a financial one. The cost of dying in North America can be very high indeed. Studies have concluded that up to 75 percent of an American's medical costs are spent in the last year of their life. Canadians face different costs especially if they wish to live at home until they die. Provincial medical plans do not cover all expenses, for example, round the clock home nursing care. Some people do not have drug plans nor do they have the resources to permit family members to take a leave of absence from work to care for them. Some people argue that euthanasia would allow someone to die before the horrendous costs of prolonging life bankrupts them or emotionally exhausts them and their families. This argument is an indictment of our society's inability to deal with this very real problem, and as such, it is one of the saddest arguments for euthanasia.

The Right to Die

There is a whole field of study called Bio-ethics that began around 1970. This scientific and philosophically-based field examines issues in medicine that are ethically, legally and/or morally contentious.

The right to die has legal foundation. A person in North America can legally commit suicide. This was not always true and at one time if someone failed a suicide attempt he or she was charged with an offense. It is illegal, however, to help someone commit suicide, and that being the case, euthanasia is illegal in North America. Instances of active euthanasia have led to jail terms but the majority of recorded cases have led to probation or dismissals.

The question of the right to die becomes dangerously complicated when the person dying is unable to express her or his own wishes: a person in an irreversible coma, a child severely handicapped at birth, a person who is senile.

A Handicapped Child at Birth

Often, when the ethics and morals of euthanasia are argued, the case of a child born with Down's syndrome or another genetic disability is raised. I separate this issue completely from the euthanasia debate because people with handicaps are generally not terminally ill as a result of their handicaps.

For example, Down's syndrome or spina bifida are not terminal illnesses nor are many of the other disabilities that children can be born with. We cannot realistically evaluate children's lives twenty years from now so the best guideline seems to be; if "normal" children receive special care or corrective surgery for a congested heart, then disabled children should receive the same consideration, as if their handicap did not exist. If the condition is such that treatment would prolong a painful existence then decisions about treatment can be made on those grounds, not on the issue of the children's disability. People live very productive and happy lives with handicaps, and, therefore should not be denied other treatments because of their disability.

In cases where the disabilities are extensive, consideration must first be given to the family. If they wish their child to be treated then their wishes should be accepted. If they wish their child not to be treated then the decisions should include the advice of an impartial committee of medical and social service personnel and family members who have differing views so that the child is given every benefit of the doubt.

An issue that must be faced is the financial, emotional and physical toll that having a disabled child may have on a family. It is an indictment of our society if disabled children are permitted to die because there are insufficient financial and emotional support systems available to assist families. The issue is not the right to die for disabled children, but the need for sufficient resources to assist the millions of North Americans who have a disability.

Committing Suicide

Many people who argue in favour of euthanasia believe that if competent adults with a terminal illness wish to end their lives they should have the right to commit suicide (which is legal in Canada) or seek the help of someone who would not be liable for such assistance (illegal at present).

Some people actually plan for this event by saving prescription drugs. They save medications which they believe they can take when they no longer want to live with a terminal illness. This practice gives them confidence in their ability to maintain control over their own lives and control over the timing of their deaths. They worry about a painful or long-suffering death or an undignified old age.

The danger in using drugs and other methods to commit suicide is that many people fail in their suicide attempts and may end up worse off. The book *Final Exit* was published to help minimize the dangers of unsuccessful suicides but controversies continue about the various medications, dosages and the use of plastic bags recommended in the book. People may use out-of-date drugs or panic if their attempt does not go as they expect.

Arguments For and Against Euthanasia

1. Pain

Against: Euthanasia, on grounds of overwhelming pain, is no longer necessary because of modern day pain and symptom control. The arrival of palliative care programs, which give people physical, emotional, spiritual and informational support when they are dying, negates the need for euthanasia.

For: Hospice care is not available to most Canadians at present. Even if it was universally available, hospice care is not an alternative for everyone. Some people may choose to die earlier even when their pain is controlled. They may prefer not to become dependent on others or want to avoid the further deterioration of their physical and mental abilities.

2. Religious Grounds

Against: Euthanasia allows people to play God. It goes against our religious beliefs. Human life is sacred. Euthanasia is, therefore, murder.

For: The religious argument holds true for all those who strongly believe in it. Supporters of euthanasia argue that some opposed to euthanasia are inconsistent in their religious views on the sanctity of life as they support capital punishment or waging wars (as in the Persian Gulf War of 1991). This inconsistency allows some forms of 'murder' but not others. Different religions have different views. For example, Pope Pius XII (1939-1958) distinguished between ordinary and extraordinary measures in prolonging life. Ordinary means whatever patients can obtain and undergo without imposing an excessive burden on themselves or others. So in some circumstances, passive euthanasia through omission of treatment is theologically acceptable in the Roman Catholic Church.

The religious argument is also not acceptable to people who do not believe in a traditional theology, whether or not they personally believe in God.

3. Nazi Germany Genocide

Against: If euthanasia were allowed on some grounds it would expand to other areas, e.g., legal euthanasia would eventually lead to recommendations to kill old people who are no longer competent or productive. Legal euthanasia would permit genocide like that in Nazi Germany.

Wolf Wolfensberger in his 1981 article describes this more fully. "The euthanasia program originated in Germany within the culture of medicine, modern intellectualism, academicism, and scientism. The program began not because it was German, or even Nazi, but because it was a phenomenon of western science in general. The explicit basis for euthanasia in Germany was described in Binding and Hoche's original work (1920, 1975), almost certainly before they were aware of Hitler. This was 13 years before Hitler came to power and twenty years before the Nazi euthanasia programs actually began. . . . Initially selected for extermination were people in various institutions who had more severe physical or mental handicaps, e.g., those with severe handicaps including: mental retardation, mental disorders, tuberculosis, chronic illness, cerebral palsy, and epilepsy. However, with the quick and easy success of the early phase of the program, and the fact that a death-making apparatus had been structured, the criteria for inclusion broadened rapidly in four directions. These directions included individuals such as: (a) the less severely afflicted; (b) those who were physically atypical but not necessarily impaired (e.g., dwarfs); (c) those suspected of genetic and racial taints; and, (d) those who were devalued entirely for their social identities, e.g. gypsies. In time, people were categorized into these groups if they had behaviour problems or enuresis, odd-shaped ears, or, very dark eyes, hair or complexion. In fact, the authorities on the Nazi genocide emphasize repeatedly that the killing of the Jews evolved out of the desensitization, legitimization, personnel preparation and equipment development associated with the killing of handicapped people." (p. 1-2)

This progression genocide might take several generations to occur in Canada if euthanasia were legalized, or it might occur more quickly than we would like to admit. If you think that this scenario is unlikely to occur in North America, consider that up until the Holocaust, eugenics and euthanasia were the subject of legitimate debate in academic circles in both Canada and the U.S. Many scientists of this era argued that "undesirable" genetic traits in human beings should be controlled by sterilizing people with disabilities. Euthanasia was a logical extension of this way of thinking. Our society already devalues the lives of people with disabilities, poor people, old people, and other people often discriminated against in our health care system. (See Chapter 3) Legalized euthanasia would be just an extension of how we devalue people now. The answer is to change our values, not kill the victims of our societal values.

For: Such concerns are real and important and need to be considered when examining any possible legislative changes. There are important differences between Nazi Germany in the 1930s and North America in the 1990s:

(a) Nazi Germany was a homogeneous society; North America is not. Any move to legalize the active killing of incompetent people would be politically unacceptable. Lobbying groups from across economic, cultural and religious lines would rise as one voice against such a horrendous policy.

(b) The Nazis' genocide program, based on racial, economic and cultural bias, permitted the society to judge the value of someone's life. Euthanasia supporters believe in individuals deciding for themselves what is best. They encourage people to write down their wishes before a time when they may be unable to communicate (i.e. in an irreversible coma). Individuals, not society, determine the value of their own lives.

(c) A person who is dying is not indifferent to life, but rather, can be respectful of life and respectful of a humane death. For those who believe in an afterlife, death does not terminate life; it allows a person to move on to another level of living.

4. Depression/Burden

Against: Those who choose euthanasia may do so while depressed, in despair or in pain. Family members who do not love the person, or who wish to inherit may encourage someone to decide upon euthanasia "for the good of the family." We are socialized to want certain things. Can you imagine 50 years ago anyone saying they wanted to go to a nursing home? Many people say it now because they do not want to be a burden to their family. "Being a burden" is a modern concept that encourages premature death, and if euthanasia was legal, premature death would be further encouraged.

For: We do not need euthanasia laws to encourage unscrupulous behaviour by someone's family. It is unfortunately happening today outside the euthanasia debate. Proponents of euthanasia agree that:

(a) the decision to end life must be the person's own and in his or her own hands (preferably written) and expressed over a period of time.

(b) the decision should never be carried out during a time of depression or despair.

(c) pain and symptom control, or the lack of it, should be double checked to make sure it is not the reason someone wants to end their life.

(d) a person's social role and relationships should be taken into account so that survivors understand the person's wishes.

5. Incorrect Prognosis

Against: Euthanasia may end a life prematurely if the doctors are incorrect in their prognosis. There is always the hope that a cure may be found for someone with a terminal illness.

For: Any decision that someone has a terminal illness should be verified by a second or third opinion. Mistakes may be made but we make many more deadly mistakes at present through over-medication of patients and unnecessary surgery.

For a cure to be used by a patient it must go through years of tests, analysis, government approval and acceptance by the medical establishment. Information from the doctor and various support associations will indicate the likelihood of a cure being available in the patient's lifetime.

6. Legality

Against: Euthanasia is illegal and therefore the debate has no merit; as a result, the law discourages individuals from taking matters into their own hands.

For: Passive euthanasia is legal under certain circumstances and may depend upon the patient's and family's expressed wishes. Laws do change, so what is illegal one day becomes legal by the vote of our representatives the next day. In Canada, capital punishment was legal for a time, then became illegal. Now we have periodic debates to change it back again. Laws only reflect what we want them to.

Over 40 American states have living will legislation that permits passive euthanasia under very specific circumstances. In March, 1986, the American Medical Association's Judicial Council issued a major opinion stating that it is ethically permissable for physicians to withhold all life-promoting treatment, including artificial nutrition and hydration, from patients who are in irreversible comas or who have terminal illnesses. In Canada, do-not-resuscitate orders were agreed upon by the Canadian Medical Association, the Canadian Nurses Association, the Canadian Hospital Association, the Canadian Bar Association, the Catholic Health Association of Canada, and the Law Reform Commission of Canada. They agreed upon a joint statement on terminal illness and a protocol for health professionals regarding resuscitative intervention.

7. The Hippocratic Oath

Against: Euthanasia goes against the Hippocratic Oath which clearly states: "I will never give a deadly drug to anyone, if asked for, nor will I make a suggestion to this effect."

For: The Hippocratic Oath was modified in 1948 by the General Assembly of the World Medical Associations and in 1949 in the International Code of Medical Ethics. It appeared that most doctors did not support euthanasia but more emphasis was put on permitting doctors to choose between relieving suffering over the prolonging and protecting of life in cases of terminal illness (as described in the Hippocratic Oath). If giving effective pain control may shorten a life of someone with a terminal illness it is considered ethical to do so. [Death as a result of medication to manage pain is sometimes referred to as passive euthanasia.]

8. Suffering

Against: People in pain may still offer us much through their ideas, perspectives, and personal histories. How much have we learned as a society from people with terminal illnesses? At some point people who are dying accept their fate and give us their insights into life and dying. Much valuable family history and caring go on during this time. Effective pain and symptom control can make this special time productive and will give many memories to help the survivors with their grieving. We cannot end all suffering in the world. People have suffered through wars, the depression, the death of loved ones and faced the loss of some of their dreams. This form of suffering (grief if you like) should not be stopped during any part of our lifetime otherwise we lose the wisdom that such suffering gives us and others. People do not need to suffer unbearable physical pain but we should not end their emotional and spiritual suffering through euthanasia; we must support, love and be with them through their suffering as we do for any of our family and friends who are growing through grief and sorrow earlier in their lives.

For: Proponents of euthanasia often argue that a society will end a sick animal's life but will force humans to suffer needlessly. Their central argument is that individuals must decide for themselves if they wish to prolong their life. People have suffered and learned a great deal in their lives. Perhaps they would now prefer to avoid that last period of suffering and waiting for their deaths. We should provide them with the support they need to make that decision for themselves.

9. Age and Disability

Against: It is wrong to allow death by euthanasia, especially for elderly people and those with disabilities. They have so much to offer us. We have not treated enough of them with the respect and dignity they deserve nor have we learned enough from them. Their desire to die prematurely is an indictment of us, not a reason for euthanasia.

For: Senior citizens and people with disabilities ought to have earned our respect and be permitted to die when they choose. They have made thousands of decisions and many have lived through wars, hunger, great losses and hardships. They, better than anyone, should know when and how they wish to die.

10. Complexity

Against: The risks of legalizing euthanasia are too great to the overall population. The issue is extremely complex and the situations under which decisions may be made are too varied to write a practical law that will protect people under all situations.

For: Some people argue that individuals have the right to decide when and how they will die. If they can find someone (preferably a doctor) who will help them, that person should not be prosecuted. Laws are made everyday around very complex issues. In the Netherlands, effective legislation has been drafted to ensure that individuals have the right to choose, or not to choose, euthanasia with the assistance of a doctor under very strict guidelines established by the Dutch Medical Association and the Dutch Pharmacists' Association.

11. Passive Euthanasia

Against: Some people agree with passive euthanasia but they remain opposed to active euthanasia since the latter involves people in the direct killing of others with a terminal illness, even if these dying people have requested the help of someone to end their lives.

For: Once the decision to end life is made, there is no moral difference between withholding treatment and giving a lethal dose of medication.

12. Refusing Treatment

Against: Since we have the right to refuse treatment, legalizing euthanasia is unnecessary. People can just die by refusing life-saving treatments.

For: People can refuse treatment or commit suicide but refusing treatment can be very difficult when they, alone, are challenging the medical staff of a hospital. Refusing treatment is very difficult: in emergency situations, in situations involving children or incompetent adults, if the patients are unable to communicate, or once they are on life-support systems. Suicide is difficult to do successfully without expert advice and assistance.

Conclusion

Euthanasia can never receive unanimous support. At present, people who wish to legalize euthanasia are, on the whole, as respectful of life as those who oppose it. The philosophies on both sides of the debate are very different but there is a common ground; most people involved in this debate want to improve the lives of people who have a terminal illness. The debate is helping us to examine our own beliefs but may be taking away valuable resources and time from expanding present services to people who have a terminal illness.

CHAPTER 9

EUTHANASIA: VOICES FROM THE FRONT LINE

The issue of euthanasia brings out strong emotions and value judgements. There are firmly held beliefs and opinions by people in favour of euthanasia and by those who oppose it.

The palliative care experts who have been willing to share their thoughts and beliefs about euthanasia provide us with information that is rarely available to the general public. Their passion and their compassion are real. Please read their basically unedited views in the spirit of learning and sharing of opinions. There is a necessary and healthy struggle within the palliative care movement about the issue of euthanasia. Some of the people within the movement have strong feelings for and against. Others have doubts. Some of the authors' comments below will have significant impact on that debate. I am grateful for their help in educating all of us. Their opinions are their own and do not necessarily represent the views of the organizations they work for.

The Existence of Euthanasia Now

When you speak to some medical professionals, off the record, they will tell you that euthanasia already exists. Well-meaning doctors and nurses have given extra medication to patients in the last hours of their lives to end their perceived suffering. They have done this, often after the family has talked about their wish that the suffering end. The doctors or nurses gave the lethal medication without recording their actions or discussing it with other caregivers. The fear of criminal prosecution is real and therefore the practice is done quietly and secretly.

A different modern dilemma is described by a caregiver in a critical care area, who wishes to remain anonymous. Some would not agree that what this person describes should be called euthanasia, but it needs discussion not only because it points up differences of definition but also because it is a frequent occurrence in our health care institutions.

"We do it (euthanasia) already in our critical care units – it's certainly not a natural death!

"The scene is this: Someone suffers cardiac or respiratory arrest, is resuscitated and brought to a critical care area. Or the person may simply have had enough medical problems that technology is needed to sustain life. In both cases no one has addressed with the patient or family the question: 'Do you want to be revived if your heart or breathing stop, or if you deteriorate past point X?' Make no mistake. Terminal cancer patients as well as 80-year-olds with heart failure, are resuscitated when the answer to this question is not recorded on their chart and signed by a doctor.

"Ventilated, with tubes, lines, IVs [intravenous] inserted – to keep their blood pressure up, infections down, breathing happening and their bodily chemistry balanced, the medical team tries to reverse whatever has caused the arrest or poor condition. Often two or three body systems are in difficulty.

"The hope in this scenario, often accomplished it is true, is to return the person to previous quality of life. BUT too often, the patient continues to fail and previous quality of life is not retrievable. Eventually a point comes when doctors speak to the family 'We're sorry, there's nothing more we can do. We'll have to let him/her go.'

"Now, if the ventilator is simply turned off, the person will gasp and suffocate their way to death – truly inhumane and untenable for any caregiver. So the ventilator is slowed, and sedatives and morphine are given to keep them comfortable and free of pain. It is recorded on the patient chart.

"Slowing ventilators and administering narcotics hastens the death process. Is this euthanasia, active or passive? Is it negotiated death? In such a situation the freedom from physical distress is good palliative care. But can death be called comfortable when the patient is prevented and has been for some time, from speaking because of tubes? To say that palliative care is not needed in our critical care areas is nonsense. The stress on staff and families is horrendous.

"Such termination of treatment and life is assisted euthanasia and in such circumstances, a humane death cannot be accomplished in any other way. It is certainly ethical. Is it legal? Doctors and nurses have responded with a firm 'yes' and 'no' to this question.

"The fact remains that technological interventions that prolong death instead of supporting life are easy today. They are too often used in place of the difficult conversations around patients' wishes as they approach the end of life. And in a society that is stressed for every health care dollar, a society where homelessness increases in our cities, they are expensive. A bed alone in a critical care area is upwards of $2,000 per day.

"It is time for open discussion about what can occur and for public education about the issues of not only palliative care as opposed to euthanasia, but also natural versus contrived death. Difficult conversations need to be had with family members, family physicians and the doctors who admit us to our hospitals.

"And let us acknowledge that we do euthanasia, or something very close to it. Let us make sure that good palliative care and comfort management are available to all (even in critical care units). Then let us see if nurse and physician-assisted euthanasia still needs to be discussed."

Palliative Care Experts in Favour of Limited Euthanasia

There are many people in Canada who believe in euthanasia. In a 1991 Gallup Canada (reported in Toronto Star, November 7, 1991) poll 75% of people of the 1,022 interviewed favoured euthanasia. The question asked them was "When a person has an incurable disease that causes great suffering, do you think that competent doctors should be allowed by law to end the patient's life through mercy killing, if the patient has made a formal request in writing?" Some people would argue that the question is misleading because good palliative care would mean that the vast majority of people will not have "great suffering." The fact remains, however, that in 1968 only 45% of Canadians favoured euthanasia under these conditions and now it is 75%.

Most of the experts quoted below who believe in euthanasia are clear that their support is only for the very few who might request it. Their daily work with patients and families in hospice care speaks to their commitment to helping people live a full life until death. Their support for euthanasia presumes that the person first received the physical, emotional, spiritual and informational supports they needed before making a request for euthanasia.

Cheryl Chapman, a Community Outreach Coordinator summarized her beliefs as follows. "I shudder to think individuals made a decision for euthanasia without considering good palliative care as a viable alternative. I have witnessed years of special moments, sharing, family closeness, life learning, and many other positive outcomes of such a sad time as death of a loved one – euthanasia obliterates such opportunities. On the other hand, for those individuals who truly want to end life – and turn away from the option – then I support euthanasia in such cases. (In my years of experience I have only wished euthanasia was legal for two cases)."

Shirley Cooper, a Bereavement Coordinator believes there must be palliative care involvement before a decision for euthanasia is made. "I believe physician-assisted euthanasia should be legalized, BUT WITH STRICT GUIDELINES, e.g. patient should have been associated with approved palliative care service for 'x' number of days before an application can be made for euthanasia."

Gertrude Paul, Palliative Care Consult Nurse, agrees with Cooper. "I feel euthanasia should be legalized. However, these terminally-ill patients should be enrolled in a palliative care program, and made aware of the options available to them, so that they may die with dignity. An individual with a terminal illness should have the right to choose when their life will end without life-supporting measures if he/she chooses."

Larry Grossman, a Physician Manager of a Palliative Care Unit wrote that he was "strongly in favour [of euthanasia], with appropriate controls. Euthanasia should be an option available to patients as part of their continuum of care. It would need mechanisms in place to ensure freedom of choice, FULL disclosure of health care information (e.g. prognosis, treatment options), time to reconsider, second opinions regarding outcomes of primary diagnosis, etc."

The British Columbia Royal Commission on Health Care and Costs took a strong view on the euthanasia issue and recommended the following:

"Request that the Criminal Code be: amended so that a competent adult patient, or the duly appointed proxy of a patient who is not competent has the absolute right to refuse medical treatment or demand it cease; amended so that if a terminally ill patient's suffering cannot be otherwise relieved, a physician may prescribe, and a health care worker may administer, any therapeutically necessary pain relief medication to that patient in a dose which may be fatal; amended so that section 241(b) does not apply where the person who commits or attempts to commit suicide is terminally ill, and the health care worker who helps that person commit or attempt to commit suicide does so in accordance with the ethical standards of his or her profession; amended so that physicians may withdraw or withhold treatment if: a patient is terminally ill or exists in a persistent vegetative state, no longer able to enjoy any quality of life and cannot give or withhold consent; and the physician is of the opinion that the treatment is therapeutically useless."

Steven Waring, a hospice care volunteer, believes that "Euthanasia should be available for those who choose to end their life in a distressing terminal situation." He suggests an alternative for patients which is the voluntary withdrawal from feeding in the end stages of illness which "needs no medical assistance" and leads to death.

Evelyn MacKay, a former nurse and now a therapeutic touch practitioner and a palliative care volunteer and teacher, examines a patient's rights to make decisions and why they would make those decisions. Not necessarily in favour of euthanasia but in favour of patient choice she writes "I guess if you cannot trust society to care for you well, you'll pay someone to extend trust to you. I consider that to be the basis for any thoughts toward physician-assisted euthanasia. The question of euthanasia is so threatening, we must each of us deal with it however we can. Who has the skill to deal with it perfectly?

"Dr. Bernard Lown of the International Physicians for the Prevention of Nuclear War [he was co-chair when it received 1985 Nobel Peace Prize] was asked how he had been able to work so closely with the Soviets [the other co-chair] when their ideology was so different from his. He replied, 'I decided I could be self-righteous or effective'. I keep this in mind with each dying person I attend. It is important to set aside my own beliefs to honour theirs. After all, their life is at risk, not mine. Their beliefs will sustain them, not mine. What else will serve them as they lose physical control? What else, through fear and pain and extremity, can comfort? Only their beliefs. And who else speaks to them of acceptance at that moment except the one who is physically at the bedside. If it is me, I don't need to approve. I MUST try to accept. Maybe the issue of euthanasia will be no different. Maybe this tool of Dr. Lown can allow both the client and me some degree of comfort. I would not think of dictating other aspects of a client's life. I cannot dictate his ending of it. The choice must be his. The acceptance of his choice must be mine.

"I don't know what the answer SHOULD be – I am not so good at 'shoulds'. The person who decides after careful consideration, to end their life likely has more courage than most of us. Given the choice, most of us would muddle through and whine a lot! I guess if Creation gave us a mind, or lent us one, we must be able to think or feel our way through this. But the deliberate act – not the sudden selfishness of a thoughtless suicide – deserves some consideration. To throw oneself so dramatically into the unknown and trust the arms of the COSMOS for support! – what a trust!"

Marilynne Seguin, a former nurse and now Executive Director of Dying With Dignity wrote that there will always be people who will choose to end their life by euthanasia. "Experience emphasizes the fact that while many people wish to explore this option, few find it necessary to exercise it. The truly critical element is that every person has a right and must be fully informed of all aspects of their health condition including a full disclosure of a realistic prognosis, so that they may make a decision in a calm reasoned way. Prolonging death is not the decision that needs to be made, but rather living with some sense of enjoyment, integrity and control. 'Life at all costs' is not the choice of many persons, but life yes, as long as there is a reasonable expectation of enjoyable participation in that life.

"When this option becomes unrealistic or irrational in the mind of the sufferer, there must be an openness on the part of caregivers to discuss euthanasia – a good death. . . . For the ultimate decision to live or to die is the prerogative of each patient/person. Once this decision is made it is the obligation of the health care worker to support and assist expeditiously and gracefully to the maximum their conscience and society allow.

"Voluntary euthanasia is a debate still in its infancy in Canada but it is a debate that will not be stopped – nor should it. There cannot be a sense of security and trust between health care practitioners and the patient/consumer unless the latter believes and knows his or her own wishes, values and beliefs are the driving force determining the limits of medical treatment. Dr. Pieter Admiraal of The Netherlands says, 'Never euthanasia because of pain, but voluntary euthanasia must be an option if pain cannot be controlled'."

Some Palliative Care Experts Believe Effective Palliative Care Means People Will Not Ask for Euthanasia

Anne Bell, Executive Director of a provincial hospice association, wrote "I think that physicians, the Canadian Cancer Society, palliative care support groups and the media have a moral obligation to inform the public about the resources available so that when an individual is confronting a terminal illness, that person will not experience the hopelessness and fear that leads to a request for euthanasia."

Wilma O'Connell, a Palliative Care Program Director, believes that "if every available resource were utilized to provide quality of life and a pain free state, I do not feel many, if any, terminally ill patients would opt for euthanasia. We need to look at the 'Total Pain' of our patients."

Carol Derbyshire, Executive Director of a community hospice, agrees. "I am not an advocate of euthanasia. I feel hospice care came about as an alternative to euthanasia. I would rather work harder at creating new ways of helping patients to address their total pain than to encourage legalizing euthanasia."

Dr. Elizabeth Latimer, Director of a regional palliative care program, asks us to look at who really wants euthanasia. In her article "Euthanasia: A Physician's Reflections" she writes: "It seems that the greatest lobby for euthanasia comes from a group that can best be termed 'the worried well'. Sick and dying people rarely request euthanasia, as the experience of those caring for the dying in palliative care or hospice will confirm. This is particularly true when they and their families receive intensive support of a physical, psychological, and spiritual nature.... [A patient's sense of] desirability of an earlier death usually arises out of a need for release from a state of isolation, desperation, and suffering that seems without end. That patients within a caring community of support rarely ask to die earlier should illuminate what is required to help dying people.

"Criteria like intractable suffering, repeated voluntary request, and sustained desire to die are sufficiently general to be totally unsafe in some physicians' hands. Many clinicians do not listen with sufficient care to patients, particularly dying ones, to understand the nuances of what they may say about wishing for death. Indeed, their very cry for death may be the contrary – a cry for validation that continued life still has value."

Dr. Dorothy Ley, Founder and Past President of the Palliative Care

Foundation, believes that society wants instant answers to complex questions like euthanasia. The popularity of *Final Exit* is one indication of this need for immediate answers. She believes that the general public does not have the knowledge to evaluate what medicine can, or cannot, do for them. Health care professionals have created an impression of invincibility and the public now expects and demands cures for all diseases. When a cure is not possible, many people end up distrusting the medical profession and health care system and want to take back control over their lives, and their deaths.

Dr. Ley believes that the "litmus test of palliative care is love and it doesn't matter where love comes from. Whether it comes from marriage and relationships, good friends, or from one's faith (religious or not). As long as someone feels they are loved and as long as hospice gives that love (even as a surrogate family if necessary) then the requests for euthanasia will decrease even further. It is dangerous to legalize killing people and that is what you would be doing. Negotiating a death with patients and loved ones gives doctors sufficient support to make sure that a patient is comfortable until their death even if that comfort comes from medications that may shorten life."

Palliative Care Experts Opposed to Euthanasia

Dr. Louis Dionne, Director General of a free-standing hospice, states his views concisely. "I am against legalization." Dr. Balfour Mount, a professor of palliative medicine, is equally concise. "[Euthanasia] should NEVER be legalized." Dr. Margaret Scott, also a professor of medicine and a provincial consultant on palliative care, summarized her view with "I am fully against this."

Joan Henderson, President of a community hospice, says "Personally, I am strongly opposed. To me the greatest gift one can give someone who is dying is a journey full of love, care, comfort, hopefully laughter, reminiscences, control, empathy and hopefully free of pain."

Tom Malcomson, a professor at a community college who teaches in the field of dying and death wrote: "I am against euthanasia, assisted or not. Legalization creates a system with rules, regulations and criteria for acceptance of being available for 'service'. They ultimately become overloaded and breakdown. The person they were created to serve is lost, with the system itself becoming the foremost important objective to keep alive. To fuel it, people need to die. Doctors and family members and patients themselves will fall prey to the evil of systems where individuals lose out and the system/social order prevails.

"The idea of termination of life becoming a 'medicalized treatment' places in the lap of doctor and hospital/institution the power to end life/kill in the name of humane treatment choice. Choice is used to indicate free will, yet I am hesitant to believe that free choice is involved in the decision for most people. We live in a society that demands freedom from pain (emotional and physical), burdens, problems and illness. Yet dying involves, naturally, all these things (as does many forms of chronic illness/problems of living [some would say life involves these naturally]). There is very little tolerance of any delay, or delaying element, in our lives. We want everything yesterday and don't appreciate waiting. Slow people (in movement, thought and response), people who will require repetitive responses (verbal and physical), people who are not clear in their thinking, people in pain are not tolerated and are most often seen as a burden to deal with. (Providing support to others requires us to give of ourselves at some cost; emotional and physical.) Our society clearly tells people we do not want burdens. [Note: a current insurance television commercial has an elderly person saying they got the insurance because they do not want to burden their relatives with the cost of a funeral.] If someone views their dying/illness as being a burden to others they may feel the only option is immediate death, rather than working through the issues and struggles that come with living while dying. Therefore their choice is a false one, the social pressure for them to remove themselves from life is overwhelming.

"The issue of assisted euthanasia will ultimately lead to the quantifying of the value of human life, which is inherently of value. This will happen because doctors will need rules to allow them to decide when someone's request is valid and when it might indicate another issue, i.e. mental disturbance, in which case the assistance will not be given and, indeed, heroic efforts to save the person might be made. Once rules are laid down the possibility of taking them and applying them to groups who may meet them, but are not 'dying' is simply to tempting. History shows the slippery slope here to be reality and that is simply unacceptable.

"The problem is that we can not come up with an answer because once we do it tends to become institutionalized and the person is once again sacrificed to the system. Perhaps we should then continue forever the struggle of this issue and fail to arrive at a systematic end point, in order to care, filled with hope, for the person we love while they are dying."

David J. Roy, Director of the Center for Bioethics at the Clinical Research Institute of Montreal has written some of the most convincing and extensive arguments on the subject of euthanasia. I am quoting from two of his articles (See Bibliography) which give us some of the history around this debate and some consideration that are not as often talked about in the debate for or against euthanasia. Portions of the articles have been deleted or shortened but the quotes are directly from the articles:

"Those who plead for a legalization or decriminalization of euthanasia would justify a doctor's deliberate termination of a suffering dying person's life by appeal to the [ethical] principle of autonomy. That principle means that a patient's informed, stable, and clearly expressed will should be respected.

"The Law Reform Commission of Canada honours that principle when it recommends that the Criminal Code of Canada be amended to prohibit any relevant paragraph of the code from being interpreted as requiring a physician to continue to administer or to undertake medical treatment against the expressed wishes of the person for whom such treatment is intended. Those who favour legalization of voluntary euthanasia emphasize that doctors are not assuming the authority to terminate a patient's life. That authority is rather bestowed upon a doctor by a patient seeking release from intolerable suffering.

"However the principle of autonomy is not absolute. The right to command respect for, and compliance with, one's will ends where community peril begins. And the legalization of physician-administered euthanasia would open the door to peril. If euthanasia were legally and socially acceptable, subtle or not so subtle pressure on people to choose this option would hardly be reprehensible. Some would then be persuaded to die before their time and before they are ready. If voluntary euthanasia were to be legalized, could we really expect that the prohibition of involuntary euthanasia would be maintained? If some harbour that expectation, then we must ask, on the basis of what arguments or reasons that would not in time, mostly likely in all too short a time, come to appear utterly arbitrary and unpersuasive? At a time when universal health insurance is straining everyone's pockets and budgets, would not legally and societally acceptable euthanasia be altogether too convenient? . . . the civilized solution rests with a rapid implementation of programs of palliative medicine and palliative care, not with resignation to pressures for euthanasia. . . . Patients have a right to demand release from pain; and physicians have a responsibility to master the methods of pain control and to administer the analgesic dosages necessary to control pain. There are recent reports that patients still do die in agony. These are the events of suffering that fan the flames of pleas for euthanasia and for help in committing suicide.

"The challenge of civilization to our societies at the end of this decade is to transform our care of the suffering and the dying. The challenge is not to legalize an act that would all too easily substitute for the palliative competence, compassion and community that human beings need during the most difficult moments of their lives.

"Some have proposed that only voluntary euthanasia should be legalized or decriminalized. This position sounds good and reasonable. . . . I believe this position rests on naive and illusory assumptions. It is highly questionable that we would be able to uphold the voluntary character of euthanasia were it to become a legally and socially acceptable option. Voluntary means freedom from coercion, pressure, undue inducement, and psychological and emotional manipulation. There is no law permitting voluntary euthanasia that could, even if implemented via complex procedures, protect vulnerable people against subtle manipulation to request socially acceptable administered death when they would rather live and be cherished. The position in favour of legalizing voluntary euthanasia begs for a world of ideal hospitals, doctors, nurses, and families. But we do not live in an ideal world.

"There are many persons in our hospitals, chronic care wards, and nursing homes across the land whose lives, by standards external to themselves and in the perception of others, are hardly worth living. All that many of these persons have left is the ability to sense and experience biological pain and comfort, gentleness of care, pleasing sound, human presence and warmth. Some cannot experience even that, but their relatively strong bodies cling to life. I foresee that the social barriers against involuntary euthanasia would crumble, maybe rapidly, maybe slowly, but they would crumble. There would then be little to stand in the way of changing the law, already changed to permit voluntary euthanasia, to now permit administration of death to those who no longer have a will of their own in the matter.

"Some want some sort of legislation passed that would protect well-meaning doctors against prosecution when they administer euthanasia to suffering persons who truly request this on their own initiative. . . . It is utterly naive to imagine that a law permitting voluntary euthanasia would reduce the likelihood or frequency of doctors appearing before the courts to defend their administrations of euthanasia. The more frequent these acts of euthanasia would become – and frequent they would become with such a law – the more likely it is that this law would be used as a legal arena for the pursuit of doctors by those who do not morally accept the law; or by those who doubt the law was properly applied in a particular case; or by some grieving family members who believe other family members were all too eager in supporting a loved one's request for release from suffering.

"There is a last illusion I would expose and it is the most dangerous of all. It docks in the bay of well-meaning simplicity, the simplicity that imagines we would remain the caring society we think ourselves to be after we would accept and implement a law permitting voluntary and involuntary euthanasia. The simplicity consists in the narrow focus on the particular situation in which one person, here a physician authorized by a law supporting voluntary euthanasia, wants to do good for another person, a patient requesting release from unbearable suffering. That narrow focus ignores or simply does not see what Loren Graham, in the context of his discussion of eugenics and genetics in Russia and Germany during the 1920s, has called the 'second-order' links between science and values. Second-order links are difficult to see. They depend upon existing – and changing – political and social situations, and upon the persuasiveness of current – and emerging – philosophies and ideologies, however flawed these may be. The uses to which genetics may be harnessed, or the programs which a law permitting euthanasia could come to serve, depend upon these second-order links over which we rarely have comprehensive control when we develop a science or change a law.

"In 1920, Karl Binding, a doctor of jurisprudence and philosophy, and Alfred Hoche, a doctor of medicine, published a book in Germany on euthanasia. They did not intend the Nazi euthanasia programs that were a central focus at the Nuremberg trials. Nor, perhaps, could these two eminent men have foreseen the 'second- order' links between their 'benevolent' ideas on euthanasia and an emerging Nazi ideology. But those links were eventually forged, and evidence at the Nuremberg trials established the influence this book exerted on those who designed and implemented the Nazi programs.

"The signs in our society of overt discrimination, of latent racism, and of utilitarian insensitivity to the vulnerable are too prominent for me to be insouciant [carefree] about proposals to decriminalize euthanasia. I shall persist in my uncompromising stand against a law that would permit the administration of death. Yet there is no law, not even the law interdicting euthanasia, that can match the infinite variety of human situations. That is, in part, the reason for the difference between statutory law and jurisprudence, between law and ethics.

"What should one do when a husband and adult sons ask, in front of their mother dying from throat cancer, and with her nodding agreement that the doctor put her 'to sleep' Saturday or Sunday, the days when everyone expected her to die. Her pain was bearable, but the periodic choking episodes were terrifying to this woman. She wanted to die in peace and tranquillity. She did not want her last moments of consciousness to be the consciousness of panic and terror. The doctor believed that euthanasia was the only route open to him to give this woman and her family what they so deeply and reasonably desired. But the doctor could not walk that route. The woman did die on the Sunday and in a choking episode.

"After the funeral, the husband and sons were crushed with guilt, and so were the staff who had cared for this woman. 'What would you have done?' I was asked. I responded that I thought everything necessary should have been done to assure that this woman died, not in choking pain, but in tranquillity. It was wrong to let her die in terror.

"This woman was dying. Her death was inevitable and imminent. Her life was already out of the doctor's hands, and anyone else's hands for that matter. Only the timing of her death was still in the doctor's control and he, upon the woman's silent request and upon the explicit request of her family, would have been utterly justified ethically in timing that death for a moment of tranquillity.

"This is only one story illustrating an ethically justifiable advancing of a death that is both inevitable and imminent. We need not change our laws to guarantee doctors immunity from prosecution in such circumstances. We need rather to perfect communication between patients, families, doctors and clinical staff so that, when such circumstances arise, all together will know and come to agree on the right thing to do. It is not inconsistent to judge certain acts of hastening death to be morally justifiable and yet simultaneously to hold that laws should not be modified to grant to doctors or anyone else legal authorization in advance to carry them out.

"Some will raise the objection: but doctors will be uncertain and concerned that someone could still accuse them of murder. They will then administer ethically justifiable euthanasia, if they do at all, only in fear and trembling of the possible legal consequences they may have to endure . . . . We should all rally to protect those who, in rare circumstances, know how to exercise charismatic authority, the authority that consists in knowing what to do when all established ethical and legal rules fail to apply. We should not, however, give facile credence to those who would want to generalize that exercise of charismatic authority. It is sane, not inhumane, to surround those who would administer beneficent death with spotlights of vigilance. Fear and trembling in this matter is not a bad thing at all."

Where to Go From Here?

Dr. Elizabeth Latimer offers us some advice about where to go with this euthanasia debate. "Society should use the issue of euthanasia as the stimulus to define its true positive responsibilities to its dying members. Energies and resources should first be directed to doing more to help these people to live, rather than debating whether they should be killed.
    "The euthanasia debate will not, and indeed should not, be easy . . . . I find the moral 'rightness or wrongness' of euthanasia itself unanswerable in the abstract. It does not reduce to a two-dimensional model, a 'yes or no', a 'black or white', or a 'right or wrong'. Some patients are in compelling states. Their individual tragedy is profound. To make the situation even more complex, the most poignant of these may not be patients who are dying, but rather those who will live potentially full lifespans in circumstances that they cannot support. Some can speak for themselves; others cannot. What of them? Are they obliged to go on living? Our present obligation is, I believe, to make a more concerted effort to care for dying people well. Once this is done, and the true need for euthanasia is clearer, we must struggle to find a humane response."

Summary

This chapter is full of information. What is clear is that there is agreement on the need for sufficient palliative care to meet the needs of people who have a terminal or life-threatening illness. Even those experts who favour legalized euthanasia only do so if patients have received palliative care. Marilynne Seguin, Executive Director of Dying with Dignity, pointed out earlier that many people may be interested in euthanasia, but "few find it necessary to exercise it." People want a sense of control over their lives until they die and euthanasia gives people a sense of that control.

The debate on legalizing euthanasia rests on our need for instant answers to difficult questions. There will always be some people who will want to end their lives prematurely. The debate centres around whether or not people can ask for legal help in dying when they choose. This chapter may need to be read several times before any of us can understand the differing view points expressed here. It is worth the effort. These people are involved daily with people who are dying. We do not have enough ideas and thoughts from people who are dying but we do have a collection of palliative care providers who work every day with people who are dying. Their ideas must be understood and listened to before the public debate on euthanasia goes any further.

In brief those in favour of euthanasia believe:

- euthanasia is quietly and secretly practised today and must come out of the closet
- euthanasia is approved of by 75% of Canadians
- few people actually request euthanasia so there is little danger of abuse
- palliative care should be provided before assisted-euthanasia can be requested
- we must support people's choices even if we disagree with them

Those opposed to euthanasia believe:

- palliative care, effectively given, meets the needs of people who have a terminal or life-threatening illness
- euthanasia is often promoted by the "worried well" rather than people who are dying
- abuse of legalized euthanasia is inevitable.

CHAPTER 10

HOSPICE CARE OR EUTHANASIA: PERSONAL REFLECTIONS

When I began this book I hoped I would have a clearer understanding of hospice care and the euthanasia debate. I began with the conviction that there must be immediate expansion and improvement of palliative care services in Canada. I believe we need to restructure our health care budgets to encourage enriching the last few years of someone's life rather than prolonging their last few months through high technology. Unless we are careful, I believe that the euthanasia debate will take away time, energy and funds from improving palliative care.

As the author of *Choices for People Who Have a Terminal Illness, Their Family and Their Caregivers*, I am often asked if I believe that people should have the choice of euthanasia or assisted suicide if they ask for it. If I believe in choices should I not also believe in people's free choice to end their lives when they choose?

I am strongly in favour of an individual's rights to make decisions as long as those decisions do not harm others. However, I am also convinced that we need a national consensus on how we value life before we begin deciding who we can help die or not. We need to decide how we value self-determination and how we value those of us less likely to speak for themselves and therefore vulnerable to the inherent abuses any legalized system of euthanasia would evolve into. I am not convinced that we are ready for such a consensus.

Do I believe that we are ready, capable and sensitive enough to have a euthanasia law that protects the innocent while preventing serious abuse? I do not. There is already too much systemic discrimination and abuse within our present laws and I do not believe that legalized euthanasia could avoid these problems.

I do believe that people must always have access to information about all choices available to them when they have a terminal or life-threatening illness. I believe that information about euthanasia must be available. I believe people who are dying must feel free to talk about their thoughts on euthanasia. I believe that we have not heard enough from those who are dying and their thoughts about euthanasia. Why do so few people in hospice programs ask for euthanasia? Why do so few people in Holland ask for euthanasia (1.8% of all deaths according to the study by van der Maas, van Delden, Pijnenborg and Looman) if it is not prosecuted there?

I believe in choices. I do not however believe or trust in systems. Until we have national agreement on the intrinsic value of each of our lives, a consensus on how we learn to treat everyone fairly and justly, we cannot have a system that legalizes the killing of people. We can never be sure of the real reasons for their requests for death. We can never be sure we provided all the physical, emotional, spiritual and informational supports they needed.

We live in one of the best countries in the world. We have a health care system that needs changes but still provides basic health care to almost anyone living in Canada. We have a political democracy that is the envy of many other countries. We have a social service system that has helped millions of us since its development after World War II. We have an education system that has produced millions of educated children who are making a difference in the world socially, scientifically, religiously, economically and politically. We are fortunate to live where we live.

The same political, health care, education, justice and social services systems that have done so much for Canada, and for that matter the world, have also done less admirable things.

Let me describe some of our systems. Our economic and social services systems do not meet the needs of over 3,000,000 in 1989 who were under the poverty line in Canada (Statistics Canada is used for all the following statistics). The poverty line means any family who must spend more than 58.5% of their gross income on food, clothing and shelter. We have over 300 food banks in Canada because people cannot earn enough money to feed themselves or the one in seven children in Canada who live below the poverty line. Our social services have not been able to find reasonable shelter for the thousands of people who live on our streets or in sub-standard shelters and homes. We have over 800,000 people with some form of disability that significantly affects their daily living but we have yet to make sure they have an equal share of homes, jobs and participation in Canadian life.

We have a health care system that spends most of every person's total life-time health dollars in the last year of their life. We are still unable to let people die naturally without first trying many high-technology interventions to "save them." Death is still seen as a disease requiring treatment rather than the last phase of someone's life requiring care and support. We over prescribe medications, especially for women and older patients, and we over treat others.

Our justice system institutionalizes more people per capita than almost any other country in the world. Our national opinions on the value of life for some criminals changes from voting in favour of capital punishment to voting it illegal again. It has gone back and forth and may never be resolved. Our justice system has yet to remedy the racism evident in its judicial decisions nor has it dealt with spousal abuse, violence against women, child abuse or elder abuse to a significant degree.

Our education system is trying many new approaches to reduce the high number of drop-out students in high schools. We have nearly 3,000,000 Canadians who cannot read at a basic level and most of these people were born here and brought up through our education system. We have nearly 2,400,000 Canadians who do not have basic arithmetic skills.

We have a political system that says changes to palliative care take time and we have limited resources to improve home care dramatically. Yet this same system can join 29 other countries within a matter of months and provide money, resources and people to fight in the Persian Gulf War (World War III). We talk about valuing life and yet we declare the loss of over 100,000 people in that war as just. Within the same year of that war we saw the end of the U.S.S.R. as we knew it. The complete dismantling of a totalitarian government without a major civil war at the same time was unbelievable only a few short months ago. The Berlin Wall is down, something we never thought we would see in our lifetimes. Yet we cannot improve the quality of how people live until they die in one of the richest countries in the world.

The emotional trauma of those who chose to live or to die is never discussed enough. Few people choose to die. If you think of all the difficulties faced by Canadians on a day-to-day basis – for example, loss of jobs, deaths in the family, failed dreams, lack of faith, their own terminal or life-threatening illness – it is remarkable how many people still choose to live. In 1989, 99.9999% of all Canadians chose to live rather than to commit suicide. We tend to concentrate on the negative and miss the depth of commitment to life that most of us have. Concentrating on euthanasia will take away from the support needed by the other 99% of people who die each year who do not ask for or receive euthanasia.

This does not mean we should ignore real suffering. Anyone who has helped someone who is dying understands the real drama, and sometimes, trauma of these situations. Almost everyone I have met and discussed this issue with is sensitive, caring and sincere. Most of them support life and those who approve of euthanasia do so only when all other options have been looked at.

It is not enough to say that we oppose euthanasia even though we sympathize with someone who is suffering physically, emotionally or spiritually. Should we not grant the last wish of the few hundred people per year who really suffer unbearable pain? We must recognize the depth of these peoples' beliefs, needs, and their fears. A high moral stance by individuals, health care institutions and professional associations is little comfort to people in need. There must be a solution acceptable to individuals and society as a whole.

In the past, one solution has been what some called a "negotiated death." In this situation those who care most for someone who has unbearable suffering join in discussions with the doctors, nurses, perhaps a social worker or chaplain, to see what the best options are. Sometimes it has meant giving sufficient drugs to relieve suffering even if this meant shortening the person's life. Other times it has meant withdrawing life-support systems (e.g. respirators, artificial feedings). Other times it has meant not resuscitating someone who has a heart attack or respiratory failure. This was never considered euthanasia until the debate heated up. This was considered good medical care with the support of patients' making decisions where possible, or with the support of compassionate and loving family members and decisions recorded in the person's medical chart.

A negotiated death, however, does not resolve the issue of those who want to die before their illness causes what they think is unbearable suffering. A negotiated death does not cover situations of chronic illness or when people fear loosing their minds (e.g. in Alzheimer's Disease). What to do in these situations?

The struggle within me between an individual's right to choose and my fear of serious abuses within our already flawed health care and social services systems prevents me from believing that we can legislate compassionate euthanasia. Even if we trusted the professionals and volunteers in palliative care who have struggled with this issue for much of their lives to provide compassionate euthanasia in the 1990s, I would not trust second and third generation caregivers who have been brought up within a system that allows, or even encourages, euthanasia.

When I first began studying euthanasia in the mid-1980s I read the arguments against it based on the abuses of euthanasia in Nazi Germany. I was angry that anyone could believe that we in Canada could abuse voluntary euthanasia in the same ways that happened in war-time Germany. I have since learned that the euthanasia debate in Germany began in the 1920s and 30s by medical and scientific people to improve the natural order of human development and to minimize human suffering.

On January 29, 1992 the CBC program "Fifth Estate" presented films recently found in East German archives. These films in documentary and drama formats were designed to help the general public and health care providers feel comfortable with the thought of euthanasia. The films presented people with physical and mental disabilities, others with mental illness, and those with chronic illness (e.g. multiple sclerosis). The following are some quotes from these films.

About people with physical and mental disabilities: "Every reasonable person would prefer death to such an existence." About people with chronic illness or mental illness: "These people should have deliverance through death." Their lives were considered and labelled "life unworthy of life." "An existence without life." As one scripted observer said "I'd rather be dead than have to live here."

How often have we walked into a chronic care hospital or nursing home and thought similar thoughts about some of the people we saw? How often have we seen someone with a disability and thought, "I couldn't live like that." As Dr. Elizabeth Latimer asked us, "Who is proposing legalized euthanasia?" Are they what she called the "worried well" who believe that in similar circumstances to someone they see they would choose to be dead? How many people who have a life-threatening or terminal illness really do ask to die versus the number of "worried well" who advocate legalizing euthanasia?

One film compared the natural selection of stronger animals over weaker ones to the natural selection that humans should do to strengthen the human race. Lives that were considered unproductive or meaningless would be delivered from that condition to strengthen the majority of the population. In fact animal mothers often destroyed weak babies to preserve the family so why shouldn't humans? At present, Canadian scientists and medical people are examining the ethics of genetic counselling and testing to prevent the births of "imperfect" babies. In Germany between 1933-1939, 350,000 people had mandatory sterilization to prevent spread of disability. Since that time Canada has also had large scale sterilization of people with mental disabilities because it was "for their own good."

We no longer have a consensus on the value of life. Life in the Judeo-Christian history was sacred. Medical technologies, such as life-support systems, transplants, and genetic manipulation have blurred our sense of when life begins and ends and what value life really has. In this century alone we have killed 65 million people in two world wars (over two times the Canadian population). About 55,000 Americans died in ten years of unwarranted fighting in Vietnam. Less known is that 43,000 Americans died in only three-days of war at the Battle of Gettysburg (that equalled one out of every four soldiers fighting there) – American against American. In 1990 there were over 70,000 therapeutic abortions in Canada. People protest this horrendous number of deaths but do not personally, or societally, provide alternatives to the women having abortions. Most women do not treat a decision to abort a baby lightly. It is a struggle between their moral upbringing, societal trends, and their personal convictions. When choices are not provided these women face a major moral dilemma with little more than rhetoric from some pro-choice and pro-life groups as comfort. We have taken tens of thousands of people from their homes and housed them in health care institutions in Canada, many without family and friends visiting regularly. We prolong the lives of people with high-cost, high-technology interventions with a resultant increase of Canadians (75% according to Gallup) who believe in some form of legalized euthanasia to help people who do want to die.

We must listen more to people who are dying. Do they believe in euthanasia when they have sufficient physical, emotional and spiritual support? We must listen to the people who provide palliative care formally and informally. Do they believe in euthanasia as a part of the continuum of care, and why/why not? We must listen to the people who study higher moral thought because they are our historical memories of what we as a group of people once thought. The concept of personal rights versus personal duties is only one or two generations old. Before that we had traditional customs that over centuries became our morals and laws. We must not lose that history of higher moral thought to modern demand for instant answers and self-centred approach to living. We must not repeat the mistakes of past societies that devalued life to the point of mass murders.

People will continue to resort to suicide when they want to die and when they are able. Some people will find the help of a family member, friend or physician who will help them with an assisted suicide. That happens today and it will continue tomorrow. The fear of legal prosecution forces people, both those requesting help and those who may provide help, to examine their consciences. If they truly believe they are morally correct in their actions they will proceed regardless of the law, taking every precaution to ensure secrecy. These are unsatisfactory answers to legalizing euthanasia but the consequences of legalized euthanasia are too frightening, I believe, to risk the inherent abuses of any legislated solution.

I have been with people who have begged to die. No other situation can come close in degrees of stress and trauma to those situations. In the few times it has happened to me I know now that palliative care would have satisfied the people who asked me to help them die (I did not know about palliative care at the time).

What would I do in a situation where someone has received all the physical, emotional, and spiritual supports she or he needs and still asks for my help to die? Remember, palliative care does not exist in Canada for everyone and, therefore, these supports must be available to everyone before we design legal solutions to a social problem. Assuming that an individual person has received effective palliative care support and still asks for my help, what would I do?

The moral answer is to say that I would stand by them, support their decision as best I can, continue to provide loving care to the best of my ability, reinforce for them my hope that they will stay alive because I will miss them when they are gone, and I would refuse to help them actually end their life. The more selfish answer might be that I would help them to end their perceived suffering (and some of my own) with the knowledge and skills I have acquired and never tell anyone of my actions. Which would I do? I don't know.

As David Roy wrote "Fear and trembling in this matter is not a bad thing at all." I would be afraid of my actions. I would be afraid of the reasons why the person made the request. Do they want to die because they do not want to wait for death to come to them? Or do they want to die because our society has so little compassion and patience for people who are ill, old or dying. I would have to trust that the two of us would do what we truly thought was best always keeping in mind that any action to end life would be illegal and that we would therefore have to treat any action we take with the greatest caution, compassion, and clarity of purpose.

I understand our need to spend time deciding what we would do under the extreme situation of someone asking our help to kill them. I have spent many hours in the past 12 years since my mother died trying to answer that question. Before that time, life and death questions were intellectual debates at school. Helping her to live at home without palliative care supports made these issues all too real. Researching and writing this book has helped me get closer to an answer.

When I was a political science and history student I thought I had a simple answer to every question. Not having an answer was worse than having an answer I did not like very much. Getting older, helping my parents and grandfather to live at home until they died and researching this book over the past decade has taught me the value of doubt. As Professor Wolf Wolfensberger wrote in one of his papers *"Ubi dubium ibi libertas* = doubt is freedom." My doubts about hospice care and euthanasia do not feel particularly freeing yet but the doubts do free me from having "to be right." They free me to continue to examine my own morals and how I apply those morals to my actions. My doubts free me to listen to people who disagree with me. My doubts free me to listen to a person who is dying and who asks me for information and help. My doubts force me to examine my fears about dying and sickness. My doubts encourage me to talk to other people about this issue in hopes that together we can struggle toward some answers.

The key, however, remains the desperate needs of people who have a terminal or life-threatening illness. They need the spirit and knowledge of palliative care through informal or formal programs. They need physical, emotional, spiritual and informational supports. We must combine care with cure in our modern healh care system so people feel supported throughout their lives and up to their deaths. Until all of us do something practically to meet these needs I believe it is hypocritical for us to spend our time in the intellectual exercise of a euthanasia debate. We must concentrate on the people who need our care and support. We must help people recognize their value to all of us. Everyone is valuable and everyone has something to contribute to the rest of us.

Once these supports are in place for everyone who wants them, we might be able to have a consensus on the value of life and therefore a framework to discuss euthanasia. I am not convinced that such a time will ever come. If we are not willing, personally, to provide the loving support of hospice care to people who are dying then we cannot delegate our human responsibility to these people with a euthanasia law that will allow others to kill them on our behalf.

BIBLIOGRAPHY

Binder, K. and Hoche, A. 1975. *The Release of the Destruction of Life Devoid of Value.* (R. Sassone, Ed). Santa Anna, CA: Life Quality Paperback. (Originally published in German by Felix Meiner, Leipzig 319, 1920).

British Columbia Royal Commission on Health Care and Costs. 1991. *Closer to Home: A Summary of the Report.*

Canadian Council on Health Facilities Accreditation 1990. "Palliative Care Program (PCP)" section of the council's standards. Ottawa: CCHFA. (1730 St. Laurent Blvd., Ste 430, K1G 5L1).

Cancer 2000. 1991. *Inequalities in Cancer Control in Canada.* Submitted by the Members of the Panel on Cancer and the Disadvantaged.

_____. 1991. *Report to Cancer 2000 Task Force by Expert Panel on Palliative Care.*

Carroll, David. 1985. *Living with Dying: A Loving Guide for Family and Close Friends.* New York: McGraw-Hill.

Caslte, William E., John M. Coulter, Charles B. Davenport, Edward M. East, and William L. Tower. 1912. *Heredity asnd Eugenics.* Chicago: University of Chicago Press.

Donabedian, Avedis MD, MPH. 1988. "The quality of care: How can it be assessed?" *Journal of the American Medical Association*, September 23/30, 260:1743-1748.

Epp, J. 1986. *Achieving Health for All: A Framework for Health Promotion.* Ottawa: Health and Welfare.

Expert Advisory Committee on the Management of Severe Chronic Pain in Cancer Patients. 1984. *Cancer Pain: A Monograph on the Management of Cancer Pain.* Ottawa: Ministry of Supply and Services.

Graham, L. 1977. "Politics and Genetics: The Link Between Science and Values." *Hastings Center Report.* 7:30-39.

Health and Welfare Canada 1989. *The Report of the Expert Working Group on Integrated Palliative Care for Persons with AIDS.*

Health Services and Promotion Branch of Health and Welfare Canada. 1989. "Palliative-Care Services: Guidelines for Establishing Standards," prepared for the Subcommittee on Institutional Program Guidelines by their working group members.

Humphry, Derek. 1991. *Final Exit.* Eugene, Oregon: The Hemlock Society.

Joint Commission on Accreditation of Healthcare Organizations. 1986. *Hospice Standards Manual.* Oakbrook Terrace, Illinois: Joint Commission (One Renaissance Boulevard, 60181).

_____. 1990. *Quality assurance in home care and hospice organizations.* Oakbrook Terrace, Illinois: Joint Commission (One Renaissance Boulevard, 60181).

Kavanaugh, Robert. 1972. *Facing Death.* Los Angeles: Nash.

Latimer, Elizabeth. 1991. "Ethical Decision-Making in the Care of the Dying and Its Application to Clinical Practice." *Journal of Pain and Symptom Management.* Vol 6, No. 5, July.

_____. 1991. "Euthanasia: A Physician's Reflections." *Journal of Pain and Symptom Management.* Vol. 6, No. 8, November.

Law Reform Commission of Canada. 1983. *Report on Euthanasia, Aiding Suicide and Cessation of Treatment.* Ottawa: Ministry of Supply and Services, Canada.

Linton, Adam. 1992. "There's a better way to keep the system from taking a fall." Toronto: *Globe and Mail,* January 24, p. D4.

Maguire, Daniel C. 1984. *Death by Choice.* 2nd Edition. New York: Image Books/Doubleday and Co.

Miccio, Betty Lou. 1984. "A practical approach to quality assurance for hospice: The program should be carefully planned and as simple as possible." *The American Journal of Hospice Care,* Summer, p. 14-17.

National Council of Welfare. 1990. *Health, Health Care and Medicare.* Ottawa: Ministry of Supply and Services.

Nova Scotia's Department of Health. 1990. *Heath Strategy for the Nineties: Managing Better Health.*

O'Connor, John A., Fred I. Burge, Bernice King, and Joan Epstein, 1986 "Does care exclude cure in palliative care?" *Journal of Palliative Care* 2(1):9-15.

Ontario Ministry of Community and Social Services. 1991. *Redirection of Long-Term Care and Support Services in Ontario*

Ontario Premier's Council on Health Strategy
1991 *Nurturing Health: A Framework on the Determinants of Health.*
1991 *Achieving the Vision: Health Human Resources.*
1991 *Local Decision Making for Health and Social Services.*
1991 *Towards Health Outcomes: Goals 2 and 4 – Objectives and Targets.*

The Position of the Royal Dutch Medical Association on Euthanasia. 1984. English Translation by e.t.c. (English Text Company). Nassau Dillenburgstraat 16, 2596 AD, Den Haag.

Roy, David J.
1990 "Euthanasia – Taking a Stand." *Journal of Palliative Care.* 6(1):3-5.
1990 "Euthanasia – Where to Go After Taking a Stand." *Journal of Palliative Care.* 6(2):3-5.

Smook, A.O.A. and B. de Vos-Schippers. (eds.). 1990. *Right to Self-Determination: Proceedings of the 8th World Conference of Right to Die Societies.* Amsterdam: VU University Press.

Sutherland, Ralph W. and Jane M. Fulton. 1988. *Health Care in Canada: A Description and Analysis of Canadian Health Services.* Ottawa: The Health Group.

Townsend, P. and N. Davidson (eds.). 1988. *Inequalities in Health: The Black Report.* London: Penguin Books.

van Bommel, Harry
1986, 1992. *Choices for People Who Have a Terminal Illness, Their Families and Their Caregivers.* Toronto: NC Press.
1991. "Palliative Care Standards – Who Decides?" *Pain Management Newsletter* Barry R. Ashpole. (ed.) Markham, Ontario: Knoll Pharmaceuticals Canada, 4(3):3-5.

van der Maas, P., J. Van Delden, L. Pijnenborg, and C. Looman. 1991. "Euthanasia and other Medical Decisions Concerning the End of Life." *The Lancet Journal,* Vol. 338, pp. 669-674.

Wennberg, Robert N. 1989. *Terminal Choices: Euthanasia, Suicide and the Right to Die.* Exeter, UK: Paternoster Press.

Whitehead, M. 1988. *The Health Divide.* London: Penguin Books.

Wolfensberger, Wolf
    1982 "The Extermination of Handicapped People in World War II Germany." *Mental Retardation.* 19(1), 1-7.
    1984 "Reflections on Gibson's Article." *Mental Retardation.* 22(8), 157-58.
    1987 *The New Genocide of Handicapped and Afflicted People.* Syracuse, NY: Author.

Wolfensberger, Wolf and Susan Thomas. 1983. *PASSING – Program analysis of service systems' implementation of normalization goals: A method of evaluating the quality of human services according to the principle of normalization* (2nd Edition). North York: Canadian National Institute on Mental Retardation.

Yukon Legislature, 1990. Yukon Legislative Assembly, *Bill No. 4,* Health Act assented to December 18, 1990, 2nd Session of the 27th Legislative Assembly.

INDEX

Alberta; 36,37

Balfour, Heather M.; 53, 62

Bell, Ann; 88

Bennett, Laurie; 60

British Columbia; 31, 36, 47, 85

Callwood, June; 36

Canadian Council of Health Facilities Accreditation; 47-49, 51

Cancer 2000; 32, 38

Chapman, Cheryl; 55, 60, 65, 85

Clark Weir, Virginia; 62

Cooper, Shirley; 56, 59, 85

Derbyshire, Carol; 58, 88

Dionne, Louis, MD; 62, 89

Eaton, The Reverend Sally; 56, 59, 64, 66

Fulton, Jane; 21, 33

Grossman, Larry, MD; 55-56, 59, 60, 66, 85

Henderson, Joan; 89

Latimer, Elizabeth, MD; 56, 62, 88, 95, 102

Ley, Dorothy C. H., MD; Dedication, 22, 53, 55, 56, 60-64, 66, 88-89

Lown, Bernard, MD; 86

Mackay, Evelyn; 59, 86

MacKenzie, Jackie; 55, 60, 63

Malcomson, Tom; 55, 58, 89

Manitoba; 36

McKenzie, Sandra; 31

Mount, Balfour, MD; 53, 55-56, 60, 62, 89

New Brunswick; 30, 36

Newfoundland; 36, 53

Noonan, Barbara; 54

Northwest Territories; 31, 36

Nova Scotia; 31, 36

O'Connell, Wilma; 54, 88

Ontario; 36, 38, 39, 45

Oosterhuis-Giliam, Joanne C.; 65

Paul, Gertrude; 54, 85

Prince Edward Island; 36

Quebec; 36

Rakchaev, Catherine A., RN; 53, 60

Roy, David J., BA, PhL, Dr Theol; 91, 104

Saskatchewan; 36

Scott, Margaret R., MD; 53, 55, 62, 89

Seguin, Marilynne, RN; 54, 63, 87, 96

Sutherland, Ralph, MD; 21, 33

Trinity Hospice Toronto; 24, 54, 59

Waring, Steven; 56, 59, 86

Wellington Hospice; 60

Wolfensberger, Wolf; 40, 49, 66, 75, 105

Yukon; 36

PUBLISHER'S NOTE

NC Press believes strongly in the need for a balanced perspective on the choices available to people who have a terminal or life-threatening illness. We want Canadians to have as much access to this information as possible so they can make informed decisions about their choices.

As such, we will provide any individual or organization a 30% discount off the cover price on orders of five or more copies of *Dying for Care*.

Palliative care groups may want to use this book and van Bommel's other book *Choices* to enhance their programming and education through:

- Fundraising. Purchase 5 or more books for the discount price and sell them at the retail price, retaining the profits for your organization.
- Volunteer and staff training.
- Patient and family education.
- As a gift to new members of your organization.

Contact: NC Press Ltd.
345 Adelaide Street West, Suite 400
Toronto, Ontario M5V 1R5
phone, (416) 593-6284 or fax (416) 593-6204.

ABOUT THE AUTHOR

Harry van Bommel has been an adult educator since 1981 and is President of PSD Consultants. He is the author of seven books including ones on management and staff development and helping adults enhance their learning skills. Mr. van Bommel has a Masters Degree in Adult Education and a Combined Honours Bachelor Degree in History and Political Science. His list of clients includes people and organizations in education, health care, social services, government, not-for-profit organizations and the general public.

Mr. van Bommel helped both of his parents and his grandfather live at home until their deaths. This experience led to his researching and writing *Choices for People Who Have a Terminal Illness, Their Families and Their Caregivers*, a practical guide on pain and symptom control, palliative/hospice care, legal and moral rights and responsibilities, working with physicians, euthanasia, emotional aspects of dying and death, preparing legal and financial affairs, and preparing funeral arrangements. Mr. van Bommel, as a community volunteer and education specialist, advises several palliative care organizations. He is also a community member of various local, provincial and federal palliative care associations.